EMBRACE
THE JOURNEY & LEAVE SMILING
Your Guide to Orthodontics

I0122074

Robert F. Garrison, DMD, PA

EmBRACE the Journey & Leave Smiling -
Your Guide to Orthodontics

© 2020 Dr. Robert F. Garrison

ISBN: 978-1-970095-13-5

TABLE OF CONTENTS

I have written this book so that you, the potential patient or parent of a potential patient, will have the information and confidence to make the best decision concerning the health and attractiveness of your smile. This book is slanted towards the 10-15 year old population because they constitute the most patients. However, I will also cover adult orthodontics and what is referred to as early, interceptive, or phase I orthodontics for the 6-10 year old patients.

FOREWORD

Why Read This Boring Little Book?

My name is Dr. Robert Garrison, and I'm an orthodontist.

My reasons for becoming an orthodontist – instead of a veterinarian or handsome movie actor or professor of poetry – are in the back of this book, if you're curious. They might matter to you.

But this book is about you, the parent, and your son or daughter, not about me. It is about information you need to know to make intelligent, responsible decisions about your child's health, appearance, self-esteem and social interactions…of a permanent, lifelong nature. *Does he really NEED braces? If so, when? If so, who should I trust to provide his orthodontic care? How will I know I'm not being ripped off?* And more.

If you will take the time to read this book, you will KNOW what you need to know, to confidently and correctly make whatever decisions you need to make about your child's orthodontic care and decisions that you need to make for your child.

It's not 1982.

To start, we're no longer dealing with heavy, ugly, tight, painful metal braces. Every trip in to have them tightened another torture. Hard to put on. Hard to keep on. Painful to remove. If your child needs braces, the experience won't be anything like it was when you were a kid. He won't even try hiding under the bed and have to be dragged kicking and screaming to the car to come in to my office.

Not only has everything about braces changed – all braces are no longer created equal. Not even close. So please try to get that horrible metal-mouth image out of your head. You're probably aware of invisible braces, maybe by a brand name: Invisalign®. That may be what prompted your calling or emailing me in the first place. That is but one of a number of options to be considered, to get to the best, customized, personalized answer to *your* child's needs. You *don't* want to equate this to buying something off of a shelf: "Hey, give me Invisalign®. How much?" It is more complicated than that. But it is a good representation of the new braces situation. They can be (nearly) invisible. Achieve more certain results. In a shorter period of time.

When we were growing up, a lot of kids didn't get braces they really needed, either because they would not tolerate the pain and Mom and Dad let them off the hook, or because the cost was just beyond the family's budget. So, the first problem IS solved. What about the second?

In inflation adjusted dollars, **the far better braces of today cost** *less* than the one-size-damn-well-will-fit-all metal-mouth braces of the 60's, 70's, 80's. As little as one Starbucks stop a day for a year, rarely more than twice that, and there are a number of different ways to pay over time if needed. So, that second hurdle is a lot lower than it was when it was our parents looking up at it.

In other words, the first of my two introductory messages is: *relax.*

I've got your back. It's going to be okay—better than okay, easier than okay, more convenient than okay. Orthodontic procedures *won't* hurt your child, and he or she will surprise you by not complaining it does. It's *not* going to hurt your bank account; you won't be reduced to a backyard stay-cation next summer and the summer after that. It's *not* going to be a maddening maelstrom of appointments of uncertain length, or hours in a waiting room: no emergencies from broken wires and loose braces, no time out of school, and no time away from work. Not at *my* office.

More Than Just Braces

My second introductory message is: this is about more than just braces.

Orthodontic care for a child, preteen, or teen is more than just correcting crooked, crowded teeth with braces. That's like thinking diabetes only needs attention when feet have to be amputated, or getting tires checked might be a good idea after being stranded with a flat on night with pouring rain.

Orthodontic check-ups *by an orthodontist** , starting at age seven or eight, are a proper part of child rearing. In many cases, prevention is less troublesome and less costly. Even if you're late getting your son

---

* All orthodontists are dentists, but dentists are not the same as or suitable substitutes for orthodontists. Read on to find out more.

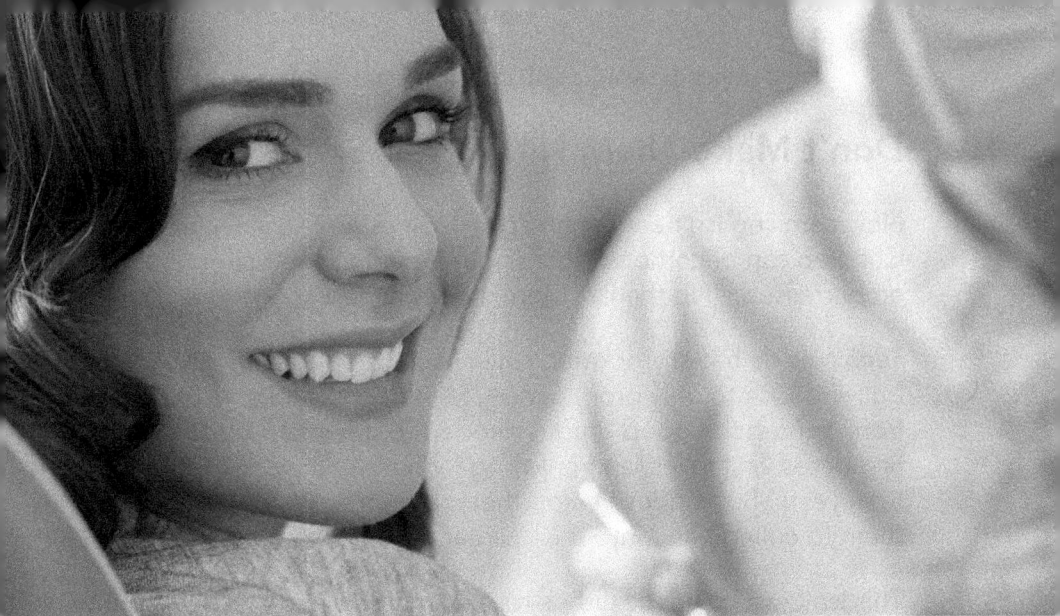

or daughter in, it's still possible they won't need braces and that other treatment options will do. But if they do need braces, the sooner you know and know of the options, the better.

This is also about more than just braces because it impacts psychological and emotional health, not just oral health. This is discussed later in the book.

Why It's Important

1. Straight teeth function better, are easier to clean, and are more likely to last a lifetime.

2. People with straight, well-aligned teeth can avoid gum disease, which has very serious health ramifications.

3. Properly aligned jaws reduce the risk of temporomandibular joint disorders (TMJ), which can ruin sleep or cause chronic headaches or migraines.

4. Both kids and adults with great smiles feel better about themselves, and that can greatly increase their confidence.

Some parents put off orthodontic treatment, but these irregularities and problems do *not* heal themselves. *This isn't acne; they don't grow out of it. The problems only grow worse and harder to resolve with age.*

Don't Make Them Hide Their Smile

Never smiling isn't easy in an age of selfies and social media. Children can become self-conscious—painfully self-conscious—and embarrassed. "No thanks, Mom, I'd rather just stay home."

Teen suicide has skyrocketed since social media shaming and bullying rose to ugly prominence. Teen depression affects everything from getting the good grades needed to get into a good college to first dates, first loves, and enjoying (or hating) their childhood and teen years. But it doesn't stop there. Uncorrected, bad smiles go with them to college and into their career.

This isn't just cosmetic either. It's also medical and can be a serious detriment to their health.

So, read this book. Be informed. Be able to ask smart questions. Be able to do the right thing. I guarantee you'll be much better able to correctly and confidently make good choices for your family through this book.

Dr. Robert Garrison

Robert F. Garrison, DMD, PA has more than 30 years of experience as an orthodontist. He works diligently to help patients achieve beautiful and healthy smiles through braces and a wide array of orthodontic treatments. A lifelong South Carolina resident, Dr. Garrison takes after his father who was a general dentist in Columbia, SC. Once he was old enough to choose his profession, he knew that he would be going into dentistry and ultimately decided that orthodontics was where he belonged. Starting his career in the Columbia and Lexington areas, he owned a successful orthodontic practice in Lexington for decades, where he put braces on more than 10,000 patients, including the daughter of former Governor of South Carolina and former United States Ambassador to the United Nations, Nikki Haley.

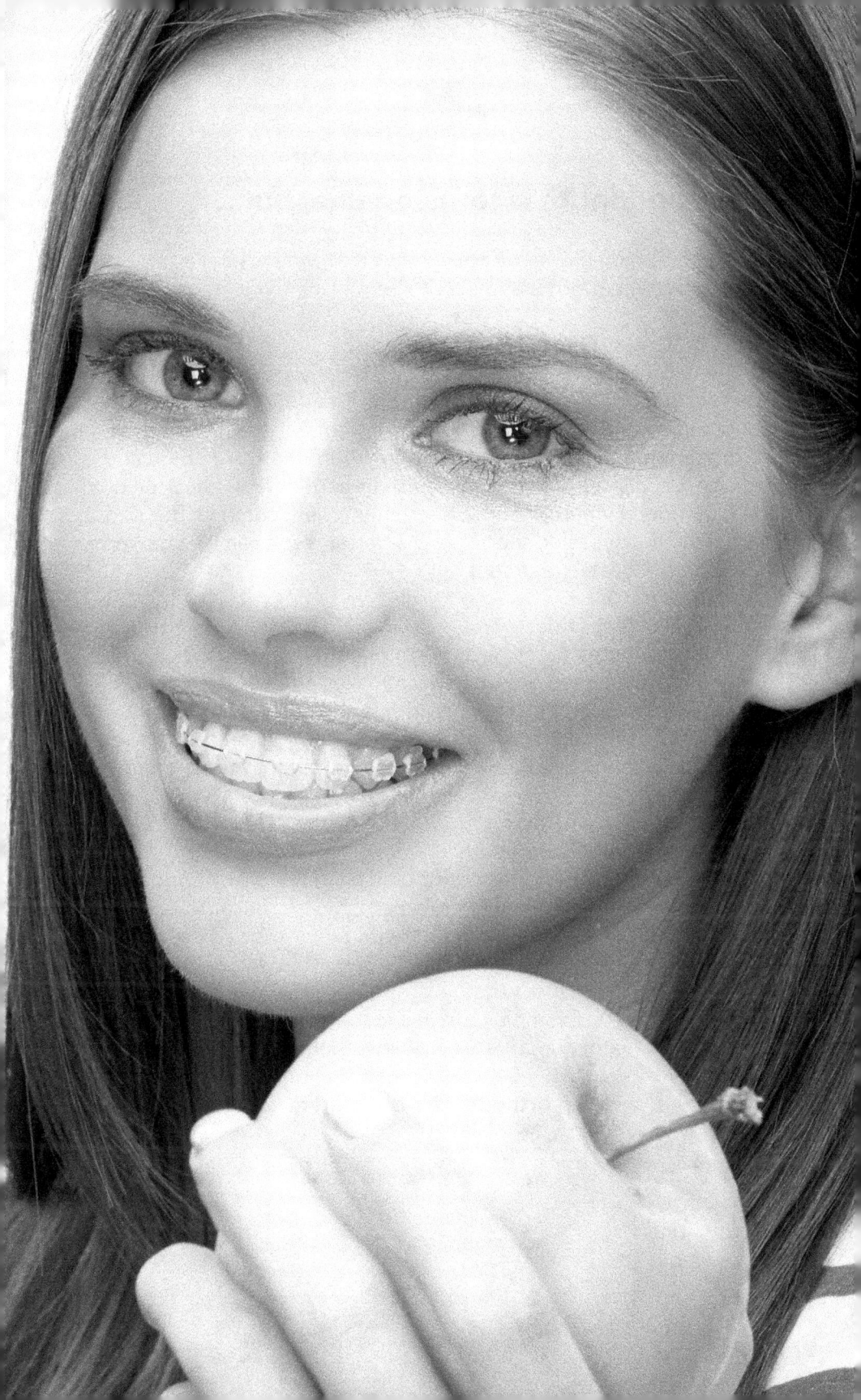

CHAPTER 1

Orthodontics is for Everyone, but...

There are three general age groups that patients are classified into and treatment goals and objectives may vary with each group.

1. 6-10 Year Olds

Treatment for this age group is called Early Treatment, Phase I Treatment or Interceptive Treatment. Treatment goals are limited but can be VERY IMPORTANT. This is not full or comprehensive treatment because a lot of the permanent teeth are not in at this age. Usually a child who has Phase I treatment will need full or Phase II treatment when all of the permanent teeth come in. But treatment will be much easier, shorter and a better result can be attained as a result of Phase I treatment.

2. 11-16 Year Olds

This constitutes the largest group of patients... and for good reason. These patients are growing which makes attaining goals much easier and faster. This age group has all of their permanent teeth which are needed to get the bite (occlusion) correct. This age group is usually mentally OK with the idea of wearing braces, which is very important.

3. 17-75 Year Olds

Adult orthodontics does constitute about 23% of orthodontic patients. For young adults, treatment can be similar to teen treatment, except there is no growth. So ideal goals are more difficult to obtain in some cases. Older adults can be more challenging due to a variety of conditions that can come with the aging process. Examples can include missing teeth, worn teeth, crowned teeth, gum disease, jaw disorders and other issues.

So orthodontics can benefit all ages!

CHAPTER 2

Why is My Child's Smile So Important?

If you are weighing the yes/no and now/later decisions of orthodontic care or braces, you'll be trying to decide just how important or unimportant it really is.

Some parents feel "looks aren't everything." Some think their kid should just be tough-minded about this and not overly sensitive. Some may not have had orthodontic care when they were children and think, *Hey, I turned out just fine. I have a great spouse, a good career, friends—so what's the big deal?*

But that was then. This is *now:* the age of social media.

Social shaming and bullying is a lot worse, a lot more common, and a lot more persistent than when you were a kid. Teen suicide is on the rise, and such suicides share one thing in common: shocked and bewildered parents who could not conceive of their child ending his own life. Sure, they might've noticed he was a *little* depressed. They knew he was being bullied and spending more time home, alone, not leaving his room, but geez, he *is* a teenager, after all. What once was a few days or weeks of misery contained in the cafeteria with a few bullies is now endless, expansive, and broadcast online to everybody. Behind a computer screen, it can get far nastier than most would dare in person. Sometimes, kids bully each other for no reason, being a buck-toothed girl or a boy with gaps in between their teeth is enough to exacerbate the situation.

Signs Your Child May Be Being Bullied

- Decrease in self-esteem
- Not wanting to go to school
- Skipping school
- Injuries they can't explain
- Self-destructive behaviors (e.g., harming themselves)
- Declining school grades
- Sleep difficulties
- Loss of interest in schoolwork or activities
- Sudden loss of friends or avoiding social groups
- Changes in eating habits

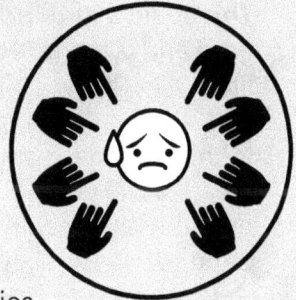

A straight, clean and healthy smile can not only give your child the confidence she needs to embrace her true worth but can also pave the way toward easier socialization at school, church, or during extracurricular activities. Do your child a favor and talk about her smile and how it might be affecting her.

Beyond that, there's a life ahead of your child. Going to junior high with crooked teeth and a humiliating smile is one thing. Hey, plenty of kids are going to school *without shoes* for heaven's sake. But going to college admission interviews, packing up and heading off to college, going to job interviews, trying to fit into new and anxiety-rich environments at a faraway college or new workplace with a bad smile—and maybe unavoidable bad breath with it—and daytime headaches from nighttime teeth-grinding is a lot more serious.

This isn't *just* a cosmetic issue. Misaligned, crooked teeth equal *significant* medical problems.

Poorly aligned teeth can produce chronic headaches and migraines, contribute to digestive problems because of the inability to properly chew foods, and make getting a decent night's sleep impossible. Maybe most dangerous of all, it can foster gum disease. Gum disease has absolute links to diabetes, heart disease, strokes and dementia, as well as, of course, the loss of natural teeth altogether. Orthodontic corrections later in adult life are more difficult; they can be painful, require time off work, and at best, they'll just be embarrassing. *Invisible braces aren't really totally invisible, and you're thirty-eight? Forty-four? Fifty-one? C'mon.*

Uncorrected mouth problems and misaligned teeth make for strangely stretched gums inevitably destined to separate from teeth. This could allow "pockets" for infections and periodontal disease to arise and turn into very difficult, painful, and costly problems late in life.

In the teenage years, failure to spend even $4,000 can easily create a $40,000 full mouth restoration case at age forty or fifty or embarrassing, health-compromising removal of all teeth and use of dentures at age sixty.

Gum disease is serious business. It worsens the risks of and heightens dangers from diabetes, heart disease, strokes, and dementia.

Ignoring preteen or teen teeth misalignment may virtually guarantee adult medical problems. If there is a genetic history of any of these medical problems I just named, you only worsen the odds of your son or daughter suffering from them by ignoring or postponing needed orthodontic treatment.

Here is what I'm told by an awful lot of parents:

> *"I had wonderful parents, but I sure wish they had found a way to afford the braces I needed and gotten me the care I needed when I was a kid, so I didn't grow up to have this bad smile my whole life."*

And what I hear from almost every adult patient getting orthodontic treatment and braces is:

> *"I had wonderful parents, but I sure wish they had found a way to afford the braces I needed and gotten me the care I needed when I was a kid, so I didn't grow up to have this bad smile my whole life and have all these problems now."*

Is this how you want your daughter or son talking about you ten, twenty, or thirty years from now? Is this how you want them remembering their childhood? Your parenting?

If that sounds pretty damned pushy, I admit: it is. I kept it in the book for the very simple reason that this is *truly* what I have heard so much over the years, and I am sincere about letting you reflect on it. All parents want to do the right thing. They don't want to let their children down in any way, and I'm sure you don't either.

You know, parents just about kill themselves over their kids' college, trying their best to guide the decision, trekking around the country on campus visits, worrying over campus culture, or taking on *serious* debt. Every parent understands what many kids can't—that it's not about the few years of college but rather the forty or fifty years afterward.

I assure you, this is the same. It's not about the bad, humiliating smile and bad bite transformed now, for high school. It's about the many, many years to come. They really can't appreciate that now, but *you* can.

No parent wants their child to suffer, either from teeth that actually hurt, headaches you can't explain, or insecurity your child may be feeling because of a crooked or oversized smile.

The fact is, your child's formative years are actually the most sensitive for his or her teeth. Now is the time to pay close attention to your child's smile, behavior, peer relationships, and confidence level.

If any or all are lacking, a qualified orthodontist may help give you and your child the peace of mind you both crave.

The Top 5 Reasons People Avoid Seeing the Orthodontist

1. Patients are afraid it's going to hurt. Pain is the number-one reason most people avoid going to the orthodontist. However, modern technology—and choosing the right orthodontist—can ensure that your child enjoys a pain-free orthodontic experience.

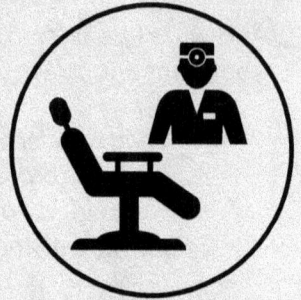

2. Patients are afraid it's going to cost too much. Not only are most orthodontic procedures more affordable than ever, but insurance, payment plans and a variety of other financing options make this all but a moot point for most of my patients. Remember, orthodontists aren't in this to get rich, they're here to make sure your child's teeth, smile, and jaw are aligned to make his or her life better—period! We're not going to let something like price get in the way of creating a better, safer, healthier smile for your child.

3. Patients are afraid it's going to take too long / miss too much school or work. Regardless of the type of orthodontic procedure your child needs, time is of the essence. Modern technology and ease of access allows us to work around your child's school schedule with minimal absences. After initial visits, and barring the actual procedure itself, most visits and/or adjustments are routine and can take anywhere from fifteen to forty-five minutes.

4. Patients do not see the need to take action. Eroding, crooked or unaligned smiles can take time to happen, but the time to act is now. Orthodontic irregularities don't just heal on their own or disappear if you ignore them. Your child's smile and overall dental health are too important to ignore out of questions of pain, convenience, or even price.

5. Patients have been treated in the past with an attitude of indifference. Let's face it, not all doctors are created equal. Every profession has its "bad apples," and to say dentistry is the exception would be to write fiction instead of fact. There is no room for indifference when it comes to your child's healthcare. Find an orthodontic specialist that offers not only state of the art technology for your child but state of the art service as well. Orthodontic specialists know what it's like to sit in the chair, and should provide every opportunity for patients, especially our younger patients, to feel comfortable, safe, and secure in our care.

Call us at 843-815-2521 or go to www.blufftonorthodontics.com to schedule your own Customized Smile Analysis.

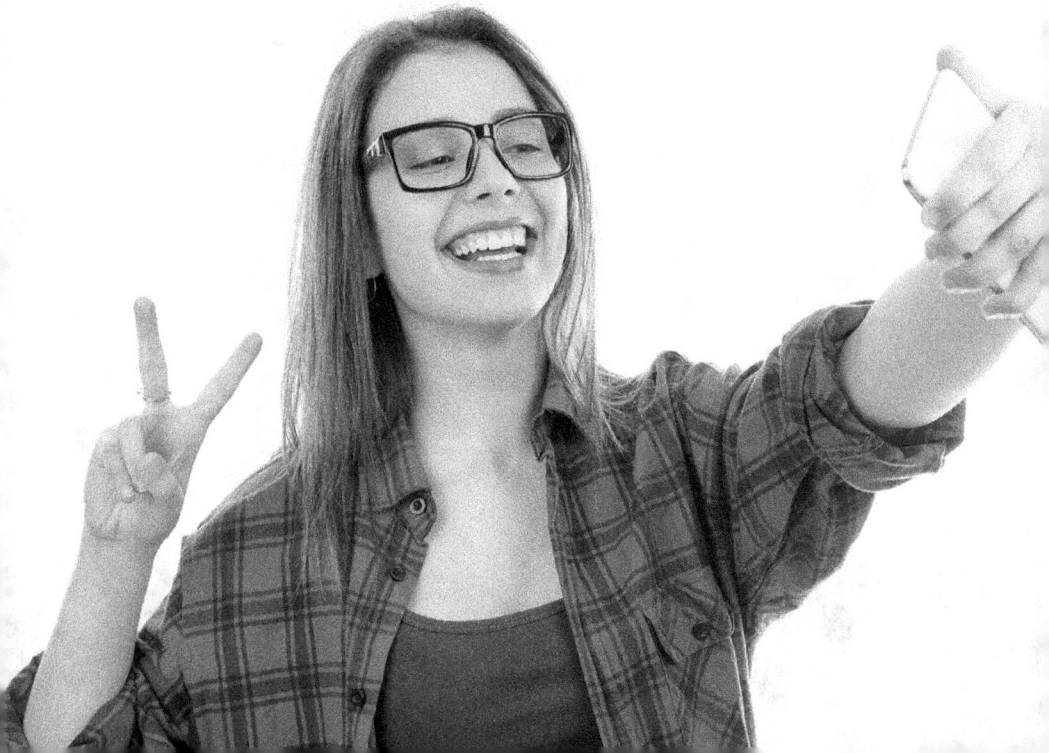

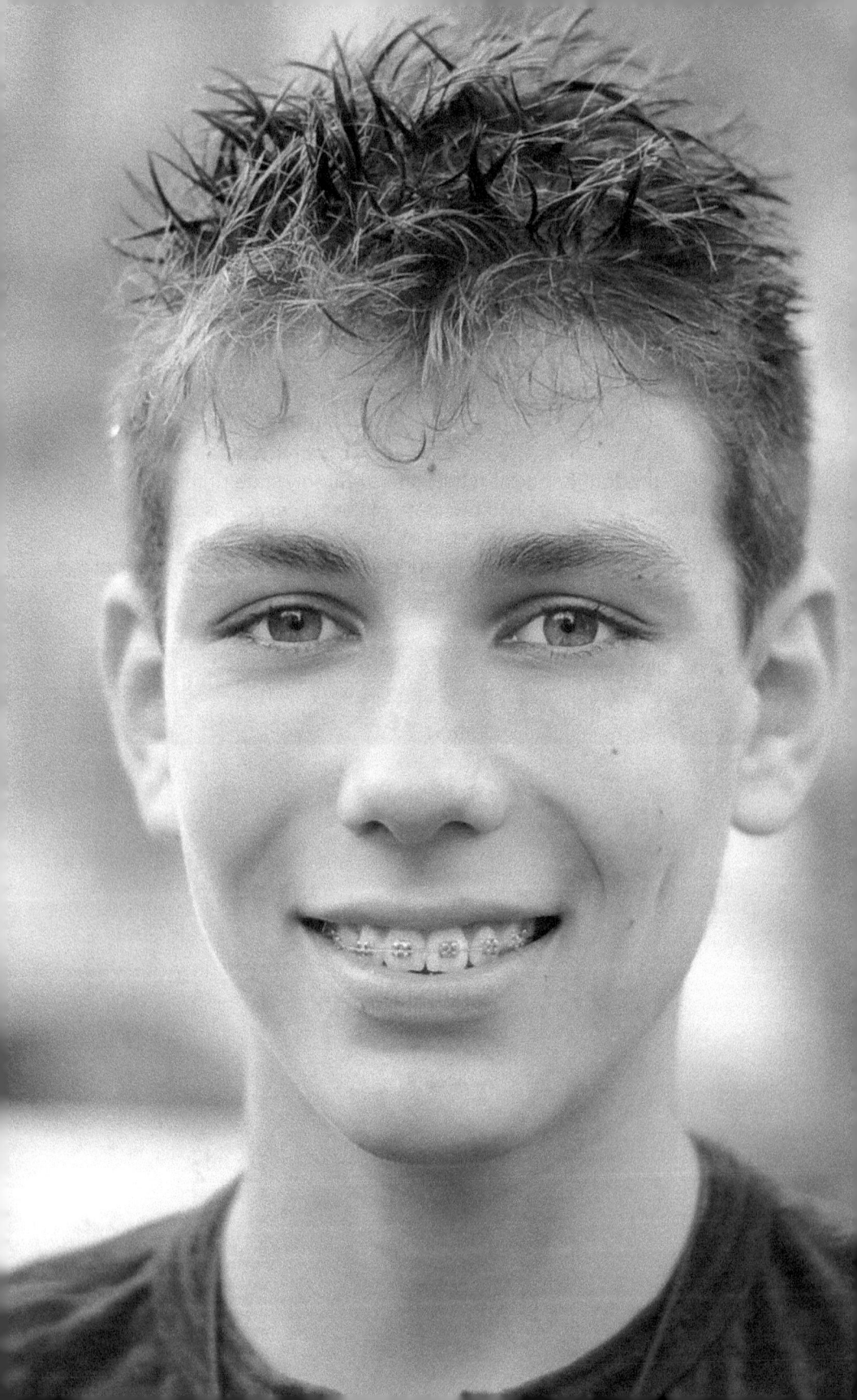

CHAPTER 3

Why Do Kids Need Braces?

Are braces something created by orthodontists to make money, like Disney figured out with the extra-charge FastPass? Was it a conspiracy from the very start?

Then and now, there may be some overprescribing and premature prescribing by some doctors. There are bad apples in every orchard. And you know the adage: if all he's got is a hammer, everything (and everybody) looks like a nail.

But there is a very legitimate, clinically documented, and 90 percent of the time, clearly visible reason why some kids, as young as seven, *need* orthodontic treatment and care: malocclusion.

Malocclusion is mostly genetic, so if your daughter or son has it, blame their grandparents. It's a fancy-pants term for all things related to misaligned teeth; teeth growing angled, crooked, and into a too-crowded space. It can be a single tooth, a few teeth, or the whole mouth. As I said, it is mostly hereditary, and your kids didn't get to pick their parents out of a Barbie catalog. There can be other causes too, like early, premature loss of primary teeth, chronic thumb-sucking, or even an accident that seemed to leave no lasting effect at its moment in time.

If your child is suffering from any, several, or all of the following early indicators of malocclusion, consider having them addressed by an orthodontic specialist sooner rather than later:

- **Crossbites:** A crossbite occurs when the jaw deviates to one side with an improper fit of the upper and lower teeth from left to right or front to back. Crossbites can lead to worn and chipped teeth, jaw pain and asymmetric growth of the jaws. Left untreated, the crossbite will require more extensive treatment later in life and significant jaw surgery in the most-severe cases.

- **Thumb-sucking:** Thumb-sucking habits beginning at the age of seven or older should be corrected immediately in order to prevent severe jaw and tooth alignment problems.

- **Miscellaneous concerns:** There are several associated issues you should also be looking for as soon as your child turns seven in order to intervene early, including the following:

  - Permanent teeth that are growing into the wrong spots;
  - Severely protruded front teeth at risk for injury or causing teasing at school, and;
  - Severe crowding with permanent teeth erupting into poor-quality gum tissue

With any of these situations, we can discuss the pros and cons of early intervention and treatment versus waiting until all the permanent teeth are in for braces. If you are anxious about the appearance of your child's teeth or your child is self-conscious about his or her appearance, early treatment might be the best choice. Not only are most orthodontic problems more difficult to correct later, but self-image and personality inhibition can be hard for a person to leave behind. However, if your child is extremely resistant to braces or is not mature enough to be trusted to care for them, delay may be the better choice. In that case, regularly scheduled orthodontic check-ups will be necessary.

Having malocclusion does *not* guarantee a child will need braces. Frankly, this is what worries me about nonspecialists like family dentists substituting themselves for orthodontists, and parents letting it happen. They may easily miss an early diagnosis of malocclusion, when it could have been averted without braces. Or they may leap to braces as the only way to treat all malocclusion. **Either way, you and your child lose.**

The first question, then, is: does your daughter or son have or show all the signs they are going to have malocclusion? Second, if so, what—of numerous options—should be done about it? Third, when?

To have all these questions answered early, the first full orthodontic exam should occur early in a child's life. I recommend seven or eight, no later than nine, especially if there is family history of malocclusion. With early and periodic exams by an orthodontic specialist, you may avoid his need for braces and/or you may prevent years of suffering and embarrassment related to his teeth and smile.

Waiting will have very serious consequences, often requiring more treatment and higher costs later in life. What most parents fail to realize is that these treatment problems are urgent and should be treated as such. If that ship has sailed, the next best time for a full orthodontic exam is tomorrow at 3:00 p.m.

If your son or daughter does need braces—now or at some predictable future time—the outcome of the exam can lead to *sensible* decisions. If not now, treatment to prevent the need can begin, and also, you can begin saving money for braces or other procedures if necessary later on in your child's life. There is no tooth fairy coming to leave a few thousand dollars underneath his pillow or yours. But if the need must be met three years from now, skipping one Starbucks run a week for those three years can make a hefty dent in the bill to come. Utilizing a Health Savings Account or Flex Spending Account can help, as well. How to fund orthodontic treatment is discussed later in the book.

Let me be emphatically clear. I am *not* in the business of putting braces on any child who doesn't need braces. My office is *not* a braces store. I'm in the business of helping kids and families get this right: get the right orthodontic treatment if any is needed, get the right braces if any are needed, and have as perfect a smile and as few oral health problems as possible. I make sure my patients are informed—that's why I wrote this book. In my office, you're never told what to do. You're provided with real information, no medical jargon, plain English, "reasons why" and options. You probably know the term "God complex," referring to a person who acts like he's God—imperious, brusque, and deliberately intimidating to squash questions. You will *not* get that kind of treatment here, from me or anyone on my team.

Kids do need braces, but not all kids and certainly not the same braces for all. Some kids are better served by other orthodontic treatments instead of or before braces. We will collaborate, you and I, to figure out what is or isn't needed and what options are best if there is a need for your child.

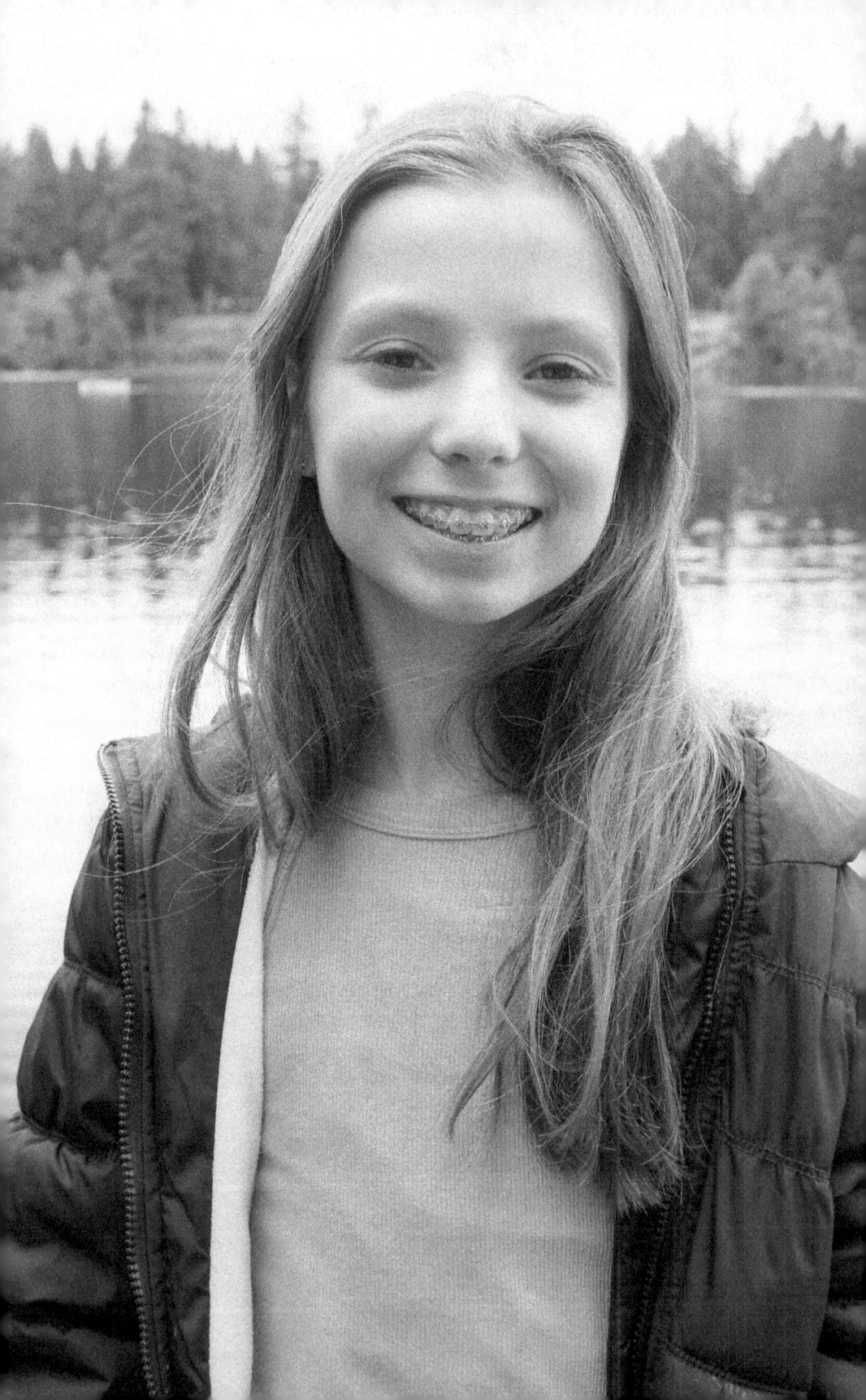

CHAPTER 4

Why Not Just a Dentist? Why an Orthodontist?

You undoubtedly already have a dentist.

Gee, isn't seeing an orthodontist going to cost a lot more?

I'm busy. More appointments?

Do I really need to get orthodontic check-ups for my kids?

Don't worry, these are all reasonable questions! It is true that, today, quite a few dentists dance over into our territory, and although they're not permitted to claim they're the same as orthodontists or provide orthodontic treatment (beware any who do), they're able to do things like provide Invisalign and other braces. This can be confusing. Here are the facts.

All orthodontists are dentists and we all graduate from the same dental schools. True enough. But that's where it stops for dentists. Orthodontists go to school for an additional two to three years to become credentialed specialists at diagnosing and providing the best treatment for conditions like:

- Difficulties chewing or biting
- Constant biting into the cheek, gums, or roof of the mouth
- Teeth that meet abnormally or don't meet at all
- Teeth grinding or clenching
- Crowded, misplaced or blocked out teeth
- Early or late loss of teeth
- Teeth grown in badly
- Teeth that protrude
- Embarrassing personal appearance due to teeth
- Facial imbalances
- Teeth or jaw misalignment
- Speech difficulties (that may never be outgrown or may develop later)

These are not dental care issues. They are orthodontic issues.

For *some* things, a generalist or jack-of-all-trades will do. For other things, you know it's smart to seek out the best specialist you can afford.

For example, if all your income is in a single W-2 from one employer and you have simple, ordinary deductions, getting your taxes prepared for the cheapest fee at the seasonal H&R Block office that opens up in your neighborhood shopping center is probably fine. But if you have W-2, 1099 and investment income from real estate, depreciation on real estate in several states, own stocks and you raise iguanas as a money hobby, you're going to get yourself a really good accountant, probably a CPA.

If you need the simplest will, leaving everything first to spouse or second to daughter may be okay. But if you are of some means and have several children and maybe also grandchildren as well as charities, you're going to need to see an *estate planning attorney*: not just any attorney—they all went to the same law schools—but a *specialist in estate planning*.

This is no different.

There are a few things to keep in mind when differentiating between a general dentist and an orthodontic specialist.

First, generalists or jacks-of-all-trades tend to work with one-size-fits-all, off-the-rack, standardized solutions. They may be limited to doing only what the computer dictates that they do, without bringing expertise and expert judgment to bear. They're often working with products from only one provider, without being able to select from a full range of options that would work best for you. Specialists, instead, tend to individually and carefully diagnose needs and provide personalized solutions.

Second, generalists and their use of inexpertly applied, standardized solutions tend to be cheaper than the fees of a specialist, but that also places economic pressure on them to do the treatment as quickly and simply as possible, because they've "cut it thin."

In this case, it's worth remembering that the treatment provided has permanent, lifelong, and life-impacting consequences. This concerns your health, future dental or jaw alignment or misalignment issues as well as self-esteem and social and career success.

General Dentist. A general dentist gives routine checkups, preventative measures, cleans teeth, and fixes cavities. They may not start seeing children until they are seven to ten years old.

Pediatric Dentist. A pediatric dentist has two to three years of specialized education beyond dental school. They specialize in providing dental care to children and adolescents, offering checkups, preventative measures, cleanings, and cavities.

Orthodontist. An orthodontist has two to three years of specialized education beyond dental school and is an expert at straightening teeth and aligning the jaws. They assess patients and determine the best treatment route to straighten their teeth and align their jaws.

If you can, you want to choose an orthodontist for orthodontic care.

You may ask, *how do I know my doctor is an orthodontist?* It's a good question and a critical one to ask as you seek additional treatment for your child's dental issues.

Only orthodontists can belong to the American Association of Orthodontists (AAO). If you're looking for a local orthodontist, go online and visit **www.braces.org** to find a specialist in your area. This website features not only a searchable database of orthodontists but educational tips, answers and resources to help you on your quest for your child's healthiest smile!

Alternatively, you can ask your doctor if he or she has completed a two- to three-year residency in orthodontics and check with your state dental board to follow up on his reply. Dentists and orthodontists in most states will be registered differently with the dental board.

Do your homework; be a "dental detective" while on the hunt for such vital information. Look for the words "dental specialist in orthodontics" or ask your general dentist for a referral to a specialist.

One note: there is no disrespect between orthodontists and dentists. As a matter of fact, many orthodontic patients are referred by their dentists. These are great, capable, and caring professionals who know where their expertise begins and ends, and do not let ego or income opportunity step in front of what they know is best for their patients. Just as the family doctor refers his patients with possible or significant heart disease issues to a cardiologist, and if need be, the cardiologist refers to a surgeon, the best dentists refer patients with orthodontic needs to orthodontists. Orthodontists are required to take two to three extra years of university education beyond dental school and additional continuing clinical education every year. They must also invest in state-of-the-art technology for their offices (not found in dental offices) —*all for a good reason.*

Even though we orthodontists have the education and training to perform general dentist procedures, we don't. We specialize.

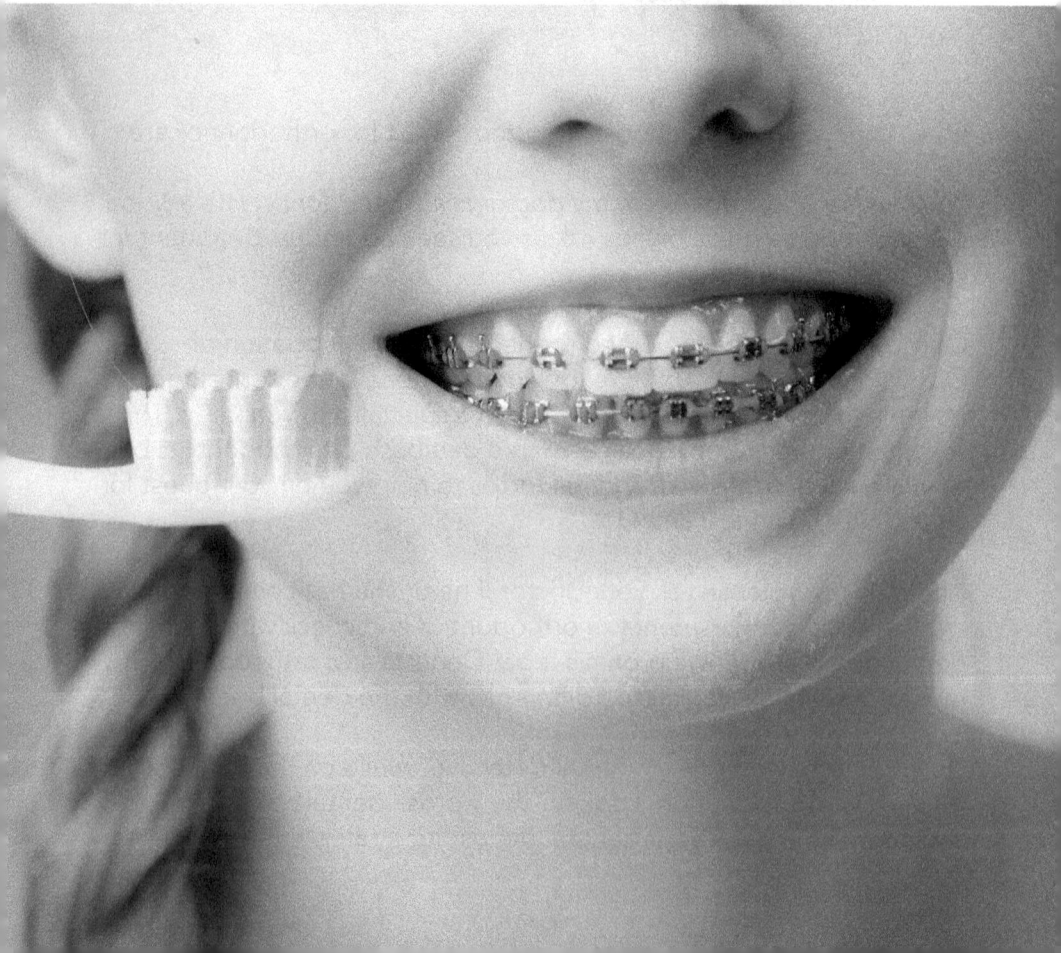

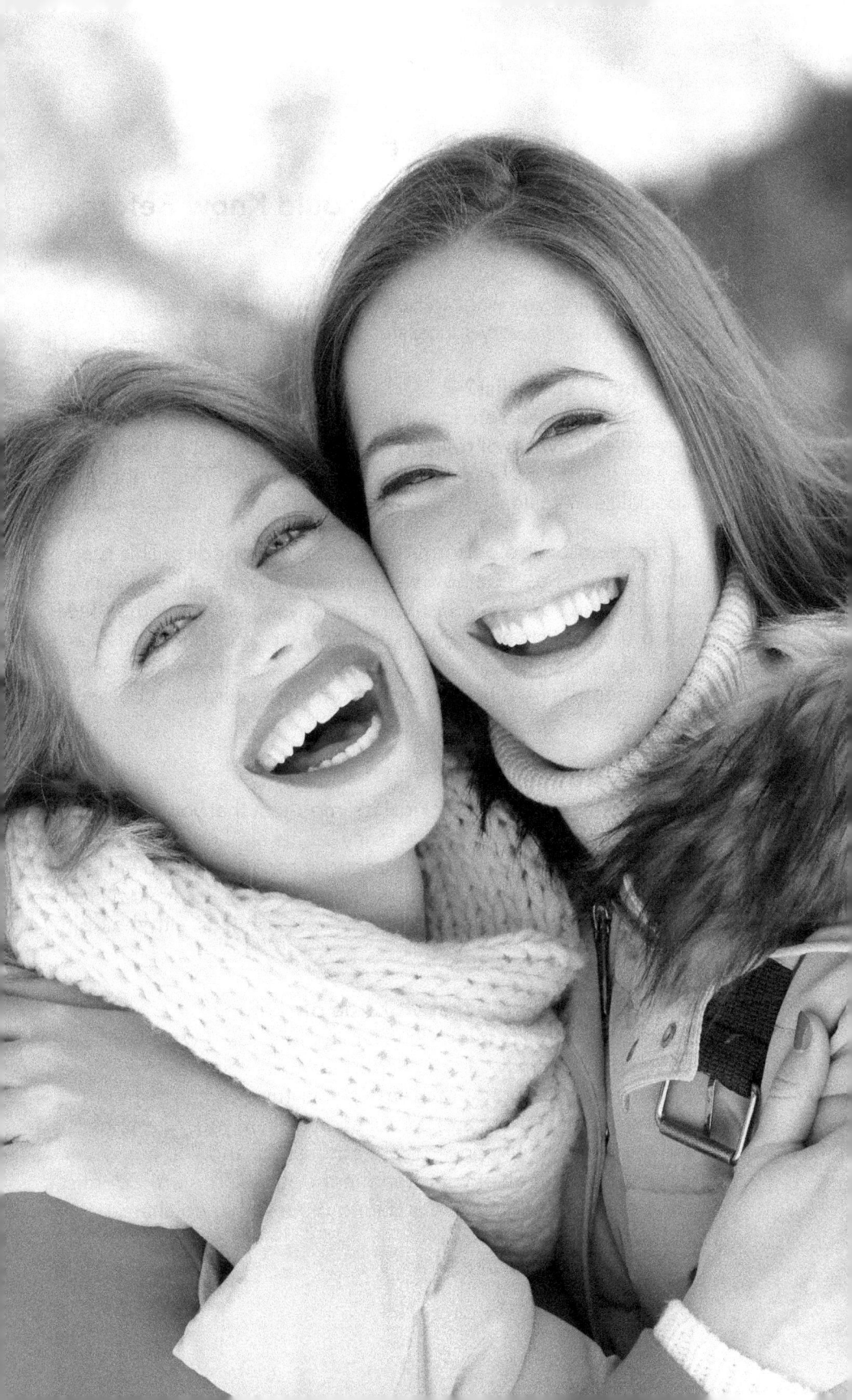

CHAPTER 5

The Top Ten Things You Should Know Before Choosing Your Doctor

This is something you want to be sure about. I've just suggested one big consideration: a very successful practice. Here are ten more.

1. **Are they a specialist?**
   Orthodontists who are specially trained dentists who take on several extra years of training in order to "straighten teeth," usually by affixing braces to the patient's teeth. You might say we specialize in smiles.

   Orthodontists also perform dentofacial orthopedics. This is a fancy way to describe how we normalize the structure of a patient's jawbones in order to repair any imbalance in their face. All orthodontists are dentists, but only 6 percent of dentists are orthodontists. Look for the seal of the American Association of Orthodontists (AAO). Only orthodontic specialists can belong to the AAO.

2. **Do they treat adults?**
   Orthodontics is not just for kids! It's important that your orthodontist can treat patients of all ages. Many adults are finding out how a healthy and attractive smile is important to their health and the way they feel about themselves. Others choose to avoid a lifetime of crooked teeth for health concerns or problems with their bite.

3. **Do they provide the first visit free of charge?**
   Most orthodontists offer free examinations for new patients so you and your family can get expert advice about treatment needs, options, and timing before making this important investment. During your first exam and consultation be sure your questions are answered, your concerns are addressed, and you are educated about all of your treatment options. The orthodontist should include digital X-rays during the exam at no charge.

4. **Do they offer guarantees? If so, what are they?**
   No matter which orthodontist you choose, ultimately you are not making a small investment. That being said, wouldn't you want to ensure your orthodontist is going to stand behind their treatment? Of course! At Bluffton Orthodontics, we wouldn't have it any other way. In fact, we offer a satisfaction guarantee. If your child has any issues or if you are not satisfied with the treatment, our team of smile specialists will make it right, guaranteed.

5. **Are they using the latest technology and treatment options available?**
   Orthodontics today differs a great deal from years past. Computer-designed braces and wires dramatically increase the precision with which we move teeth and shorten treatment time. Tie-free braces systems have made treatment far more efficient and comfortable.

   Clear braces offer a cosmetically pleasing alternative, while Invisalign offers patients an entirely brace-free option. Did you know that Invisalign also has a special treatment system just for teens?

6. **Does their quoted fee include retainers?**
   Each orthodontic office has its own fee schedules, and doctors often charge differently for procedures. All orthodontists should offer you a contract that clearly spells out the expenses for your child's treatment before it begins.

   Throughout the orthodontic industry, it's common to find out about retainer fees after you start treatment. You should ask your orthodontist about what retainers cost and also if there are any other hidden fees.

7. **Do they charge for emergency appointments?**
   Some minor discomfort may occur with braces. Orthodontists typically provide adjustments for poking wires and loose appliances free of charge.

   At Bluffton, we do provide these types of adjustments free of charge, but you should definitely ask about adjustments and potential costs with your orthodontist before you start treatment.

Keep in mind; if your braces are broken or damaged due to noncompliance with dietary restrictions, this may result in repair charges. With Bluffton Orthodontics, if you do your best to avoid breaking your braces and follow the simple dietary guidelines that we will share with you, then you should have no additional costs for adjustments throughout your treatment, even if it's an emergency.

8. **Do they make you feel special and comfortable?**
Regardless if you are reading this book for your own treatment or for your child's treatment, when you meet with your orthodontist, you should definitely feel comfortable. At Bluffton Orthodontics, we strive to make you as comfortable as possible before, during, and after treatment. You are special and we want you to feel special every time you see us.

Particularly important if you are reading this book for the treatment of your child, we also ensure your child feels special every time they visit. Since our doctors are so involved with children and young adults, we can empathize, relate to them, and make them feel comfortable and extra special.

9. **Do they have a great reputation?**
With the Internet, it is extremely easy to pull up ratings and reviews from patients. Simply go to Google and search for orthodontist reviews and ratings with your town.

Additionally, look on the website for video testimonials from actual patients. You can also ask the orthodontist for references.

Finally, you should make sure your orthodontist is a member of the Better Business Bureau and has a great rating with them. Being a member of the BBB shows you that the orthodontist takes pride in providing great customer service and treats patients the way they should be treated.

10. Are they flexible with payment options?

Once you are comfortable and you know specifically which orthodontist you want to treat you or your child, the next question is typically, "How much is this going to cost and how am I going to pay for this?" We help you understand different payment options from maximizing the most insurance benefits to flex spending accounts to even interest-free payment plans. During the initial exam and complimentary consultation, we will answer all of your questions, including those about our typical cost of braces and the variety of payment options available.

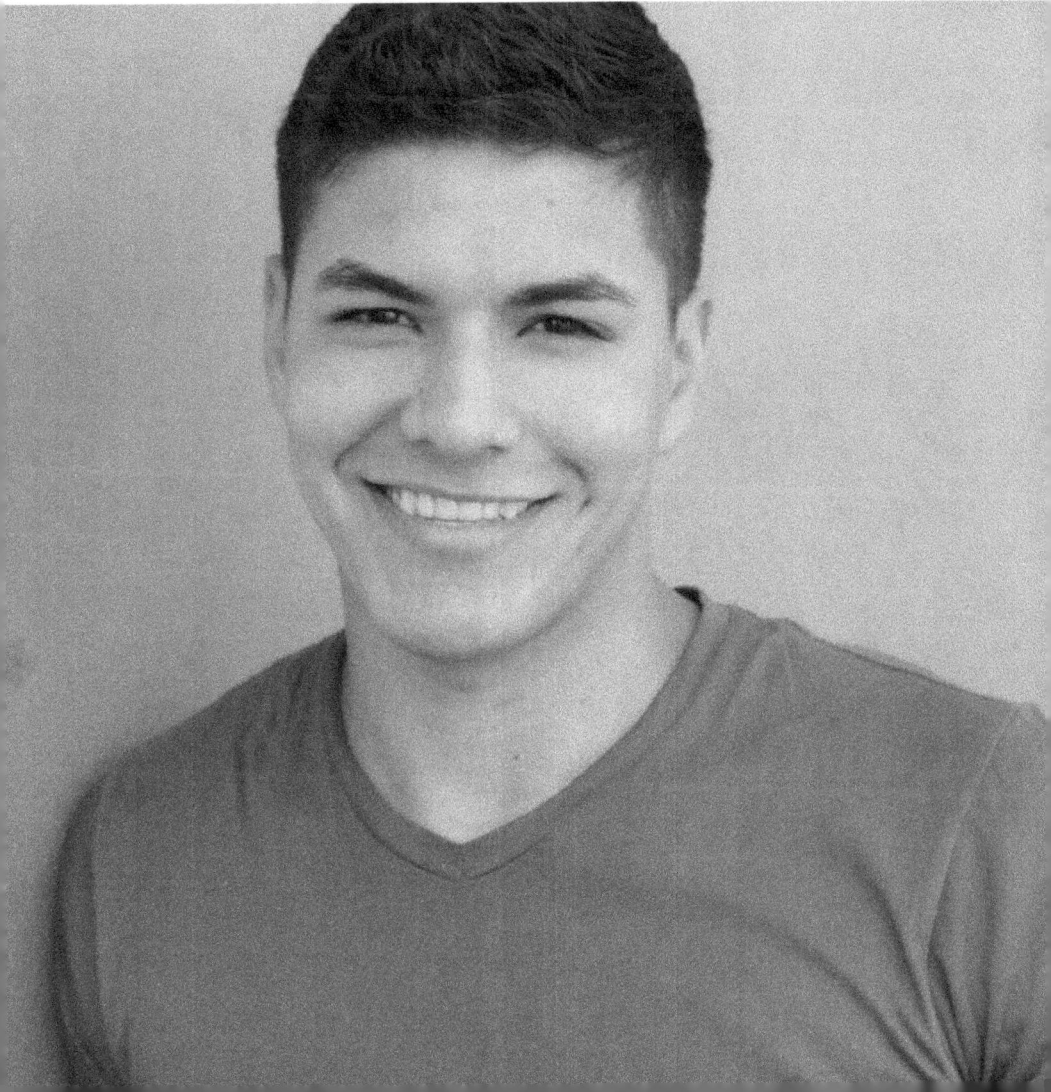

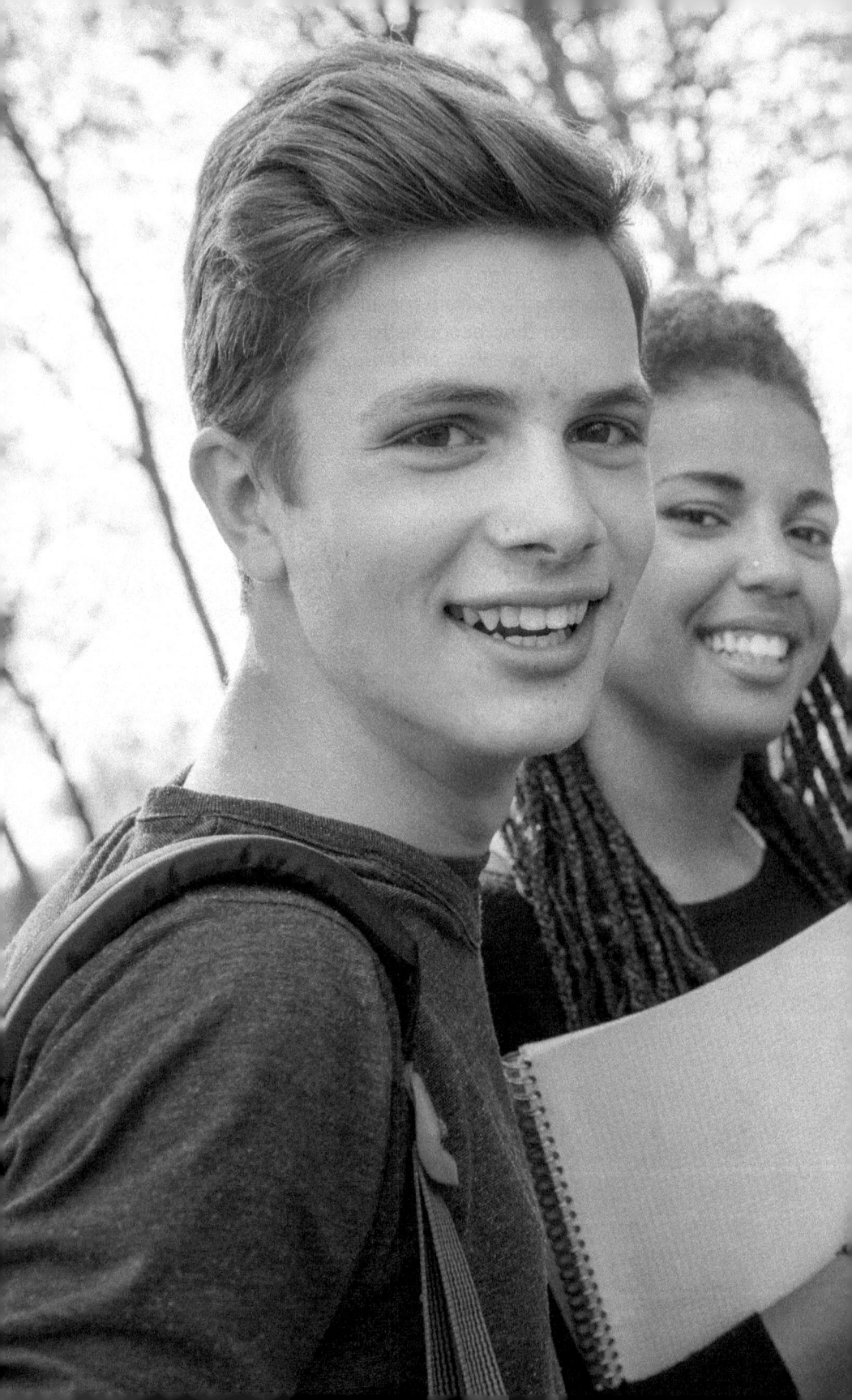

CHAPTER 6

What Can I Expect at the Initial Consultation and Exam?

Many questions surround your first visit to a new orthodontist, not the least of which is the subject of this particular chapter: *what will happen at the initial consultation?*

To answer this very common question, and perhaps several others you might not even realize you need answering yet, let me walk you through the typical first office visit, from the initial appointment forward. Your first appointment is scheduled following your initial phone call to your orthodontist's office

1: On arrival at the office, you will be greeted by one of our certified treatment coordinators. She or he is fully prepared to make everything from the first appointment to an entire treatment program go smoothly for you and your child. Your treatment coordinator will be yours, to manage your relationship with us, from appointment scheduling for your convenience to answering questions.

At the initial visit, your treatment coordinator will review your child's patient information and health history and and/or any appearance concerns with you.

This interview and required-by-law paperwork doesn't take long.

2: Next, your orthodontist will conduct the "Customized Smile Analysis," the most complete and thorough orthodontic exam, including teeth, gums, mouth, jaws, and face. Typically, safe digital X-rays are taken of the teeth and surrounding bone and of the jaw structures.

Usually that same day, your orthodontist will present his or her "report of findings," a "show-n-tell" in plain English (not medical jargon) of the full state of your child's teeth, gums, mouth and jaws, and diagnosis of any present or anticipated problems that should get orthodontic treatment. If treatment should occur, your orthodontist will present recommendations and options. This will be an individualized, personalized plan of treatment, not "braces in a box, off the shelf." By this report of findings, you will know:

- What teeth or jaw misalignment or other problems exist or are developing
- What the health ramifications are of not intervening with treatment
- What the appearance ramifications are of not intervening with treatment
- If braces are needed now or later
- Which type of braces will be best in your situation
- What the complete treatment program will consist of: things like braces, number of appointments, and average time of each office visit
- What results will be achieved

3: **All your questions will be answered.** There are no dumb or embarrassing questions. Of the countless patients who have visited my office, every one of them had questions! We do not want you or your son or daughter just nodding, then later wondering, "what did he mean by that?" or saying "I wish I'd asked about …" This is not one of those "I'm the doctor—trust me—just do what I say because I said so" offices. Most questions will have been answered by the pre-exam video, other literature provided to you, this book, and your orthodontist's report of findings, but it's a lot to take in. So, any and all questions you have should be asked and answered. Our goal is not just a terrific orthodontic outcome ensuring a healthy, attractive smile but also your anxiety-free comfort from start to finish.

4: **Finally, your treatment coordinator will explain the costs of the prescribed treatment program and discuss payment arrangements as needed.** Presuming proceeding, the next two appointments will be scheduled, for the installation of braces and/or other treatment. As the saying goes, a journey of a thousand steps begins with the first one, and a task well begun is sooner done!

In total, you should allow about one hour for this entire initial consultation and exam.

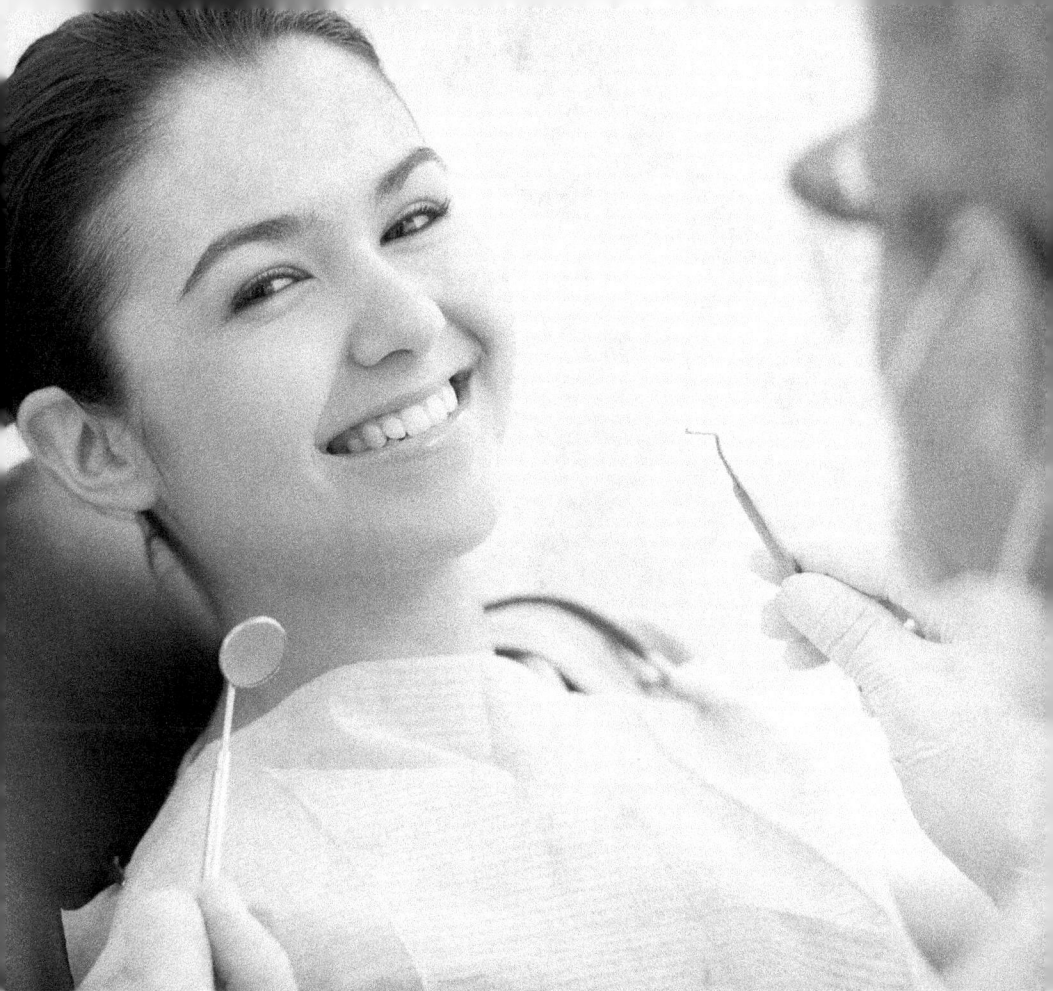

If that seems like a lot, keep in mind there are lifetime health, appearance, and personality aspects of this. And it is not "installing tires"—not if it is done properly and expertly. Your son or daughter deserves a careful, thorough, and anxieties-eliminated experience. You want to make the best decisions for them.

Frankly, our practice and our process is not for everybody. We attract and "resonate with" parents who are quite serious about their responsibilities and committed to giving their child every possible advantage in life—certainly not unnecessary disadvantages. If you are that parent, and the fact that you took the trouble to obtain and read this book suggests it, then you are going to recognize that this is time well invested in the best possible results.

Call us at 843-815-2521 or go to www.blufftonorthodontics.com to schedule your own Customized Smile Analysis.

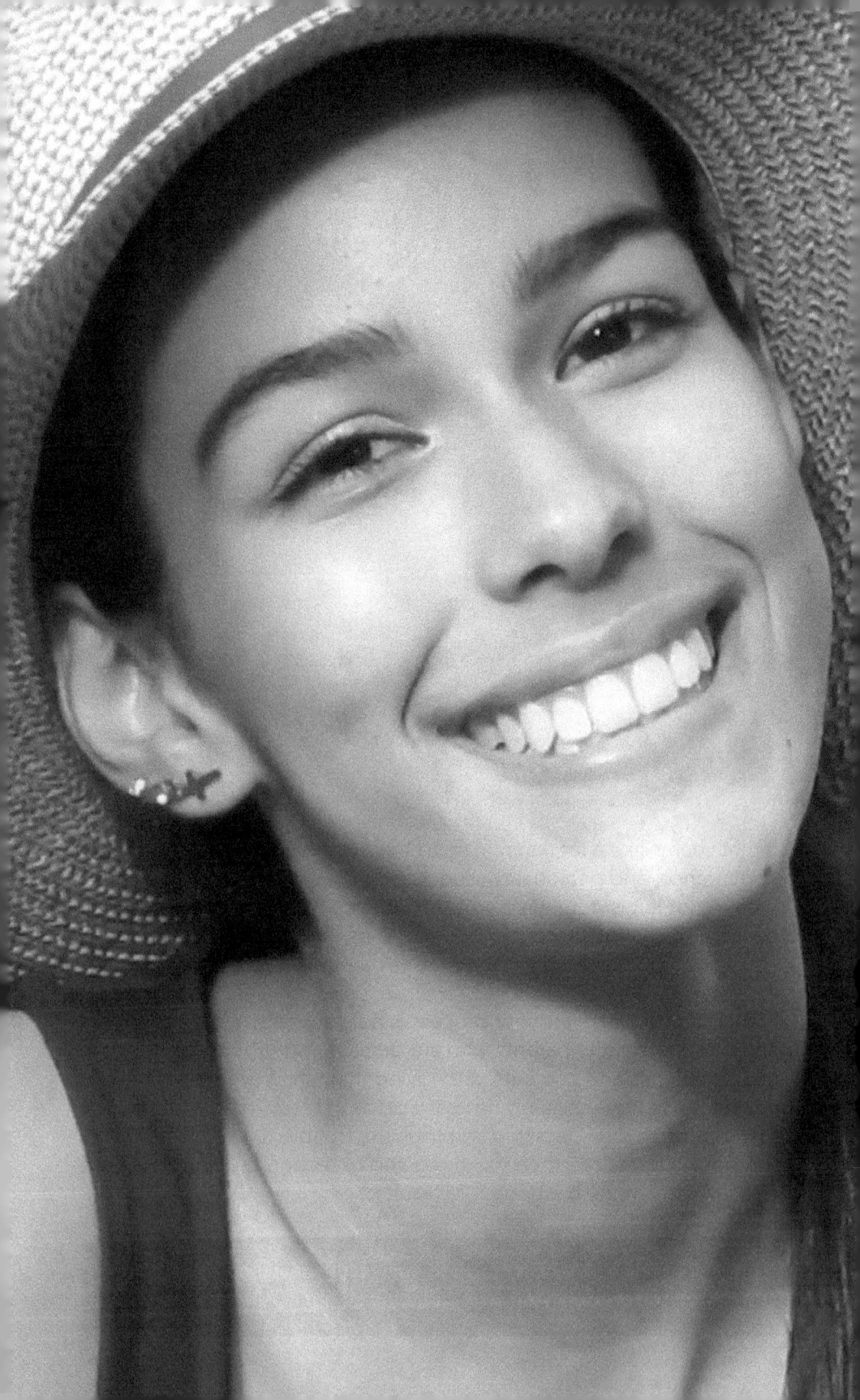

CHAPTER 7

Shouldn't There Be a Guarantee?

Healthcare is notorious for no guarantees.

Surgeons have a dark-humor insiders' joke: dead patients can't sue.

If you've seen reality TV shows about plastic surgery, like the popular one airing as I wrote this, *Botched*, you know things can go horribly wrong.

Guarantees are controversial in all kinds of healthcare including orthodontics. Many doctors are upset by the very idea. One huffed and puffed at me, "What do you think you're doing with this guarantee nonsense? We aren't operating a car shop, installing mufflers and guaranteeing them for five thousand miles.

His doctor ego was mightily offended. But I doubt you will be, with the challenge of deciding who should be your family's *trusted* orthodontist. So, yes, I think there should be a guarantee! In fact, many guarantees!

1. **If you aren't satisfied with your son or daughter's orthodontic treatment, new smile outcome or patient/ parent experience, *our team of specialists will make it right, guaranteed.***

2. **Also, the quality of the orthodontic treatment itself is *guaranteed for life.*** If ever the proper teeth alignment originally achieved somehow begins to fail, we will welcome you back and do everything we can to correct the problem.

3. **You also have a safety in numbers guarantee.** The diagnostic and prescriptive methods and state-of-the-art technology and the braces products we use have been used by top orthodontists nationwide to treat more than one million patients successfully.

4. **You also have my guarantee that *every* orthodontist and**

orthodontic assistant at my office has been not only academically educated but also *thoroughly* trained. They all follow the same proven method to diagnose needs, plan the best and personalized treatments for every patient, and manage for best results from day one through after-care. There is nobody "learning on the job" with your child—ever. All patient care is supervised and reviewed by me. We also invest in frequent state-of-art clinical continuing education for our team exceeding all state licensing requirements. Above and beyond.

5. **You also have *my guarantee of exceptional courtesy and customer service.*** Yes, you are my patient, but we can be honest about this—my practice is not just a health care provider, it is a business. As such, it has, in my opinion, one set of responsibilities to you as the parent of a patient and one set to the patient, including telling the whole truth and nothing but the truth, prescribing in the patient's best interest, and delivering the best possible treatment and outcomes. There's also a second, separate set of responsibilities to you as a customer, including access, convenience, responsiveness, and "red carpet service."

These five guarantees are included in your treatment program fee.

For starters, I can guarantee you the best, most thorough orthodontic exam, and I encourage coming in for it now.

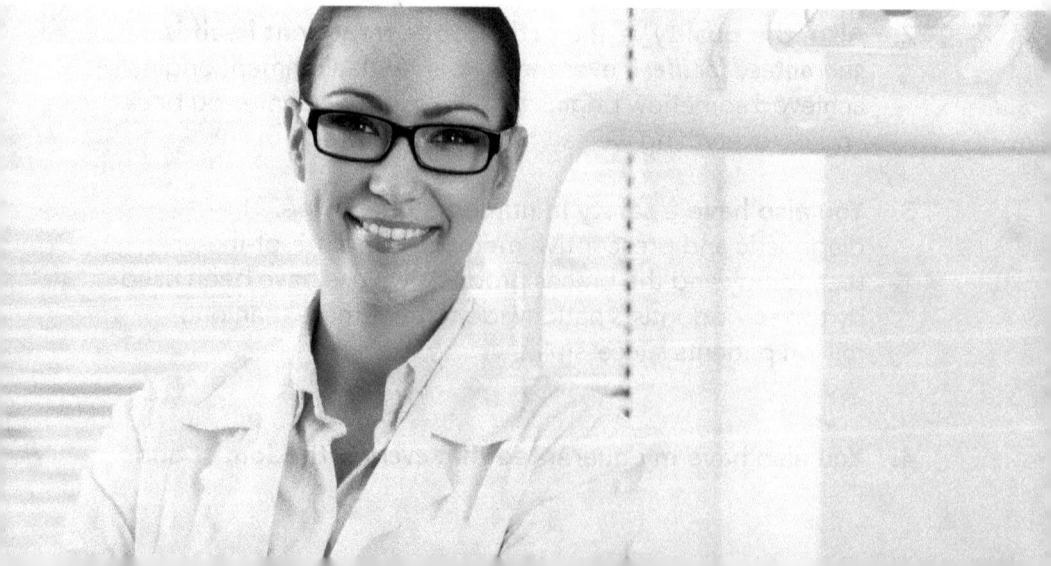

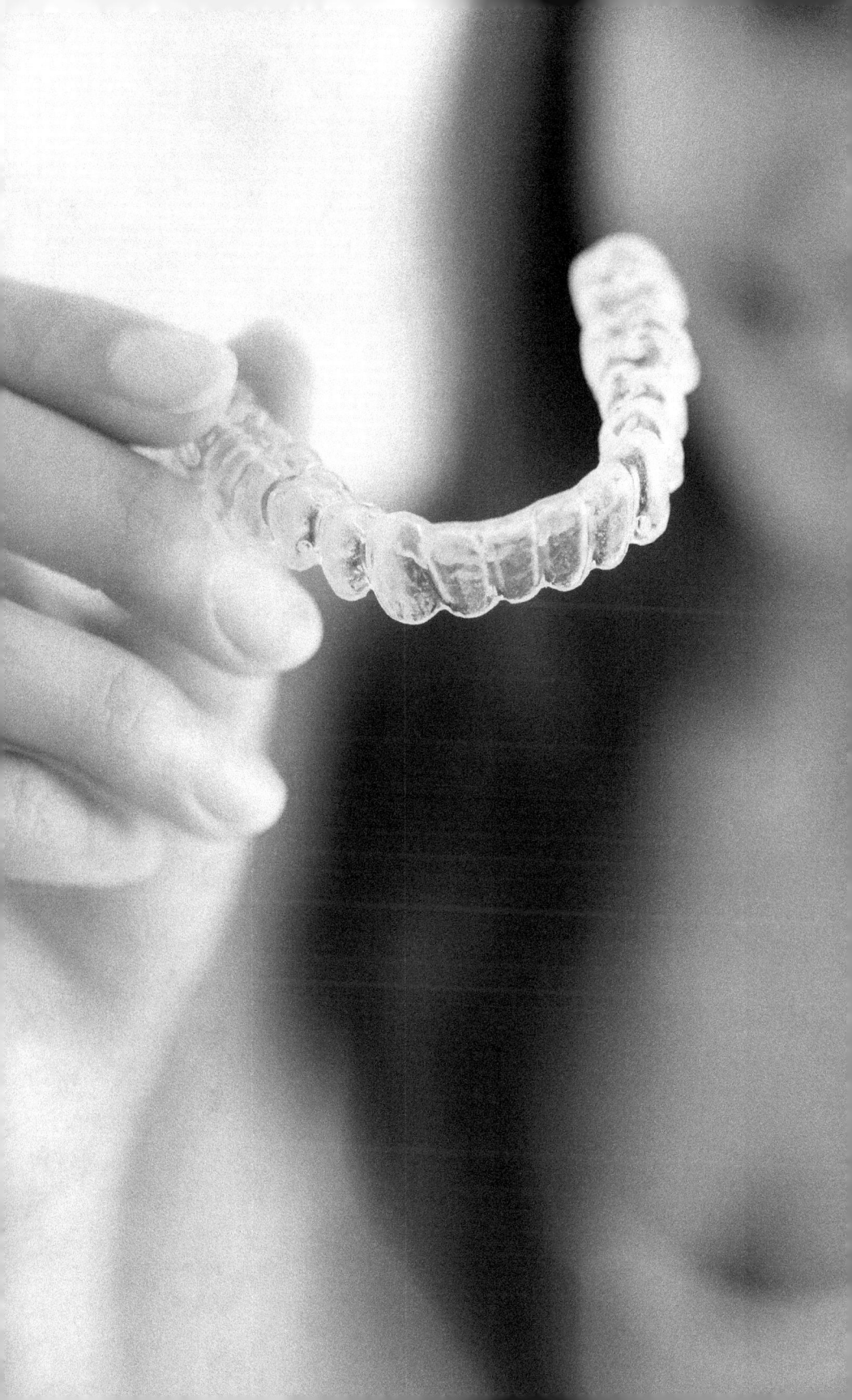

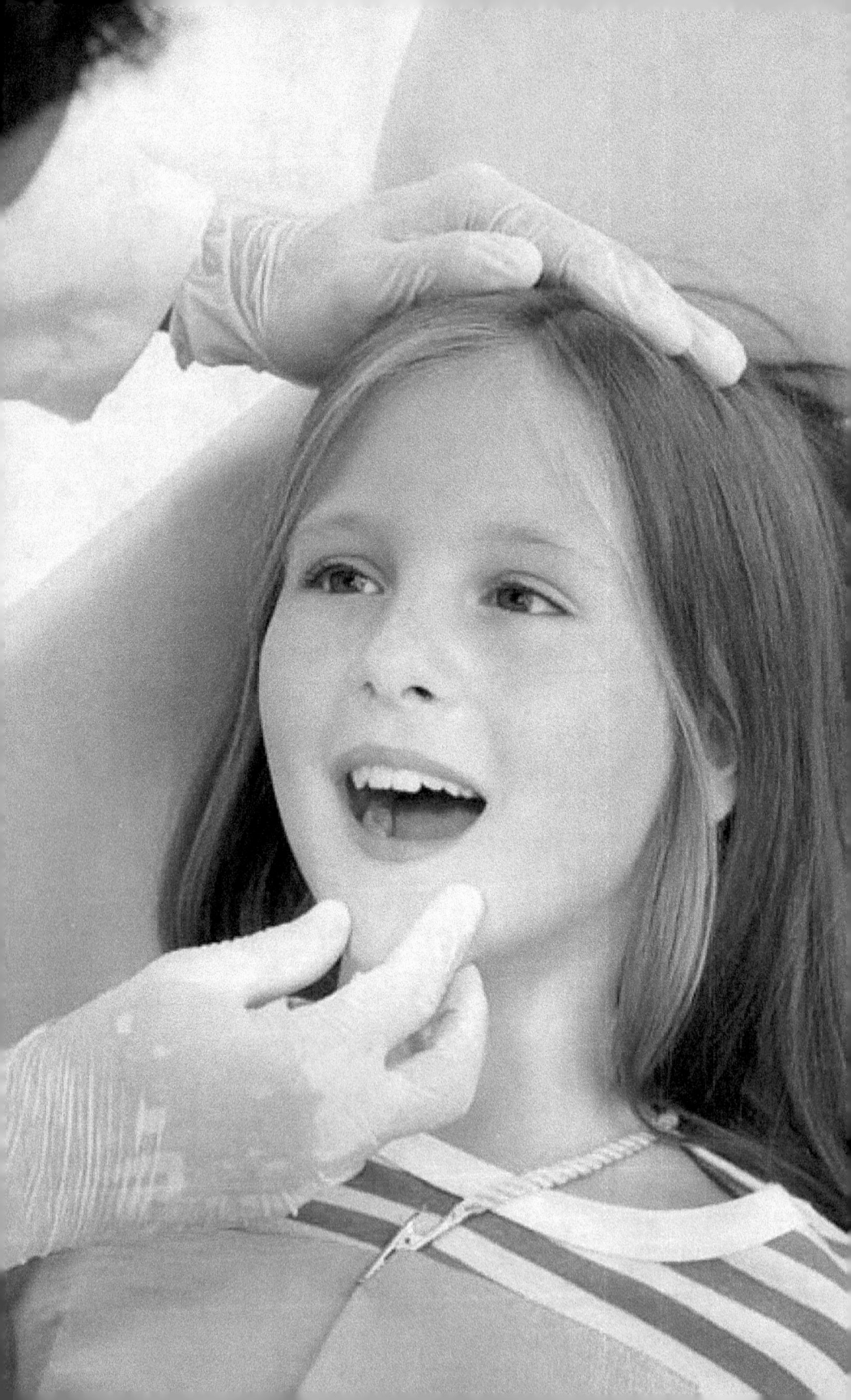

CHAPTER 8

How to Pay for Orthodontic Treatment & Braces

You may have never needed braces. Or you may have needed them and gotten them. Or you may be among the tens of thousands of people in our generation who needed them but did not get them, perhaps because your family decided they couldn't afford them. Maybe they didn't consider it a priority and probably underestimated the lifelong results of the decision. You may not only have lived with a "hide your smile" habit unnecessarily, but you may have developed chronic jaw pain and headaches, difficulty chewing, or even periodontal disease that could have been prevented.

Regardless of which group you're in—and I hope it's not the third—I hope you will be making the best choices for your son or daughter today, without being hamstrung just by the finances. Truth is, parents pay out the same cost for a number of different things not nearly as vital as health or emotional well-being without blinking, mostly because it's paid in installments or just never really *considered*, like the monthly cost for minutes/data on mobile devices, added up for a year or two. The additional insurance cost and other costs when the teenager gets his driver's permit; after all, what's the choice? The cost of braces leaps up and stands there, all at one time. So it can seem big. And it tempts thoughts of "maybe later" or "is this really necessary?"

I hope in the prior chapters I have succeeded at getting the "is it really necessary?" question erased. If there is visible need or if expert examination by an orthodontist and his explanation of what he finds and can show you say it is advisable, it is necessary! It won't fix itself. It will probably get worse. It plagues a person's health, emotional well-being, social life, and career. It can link to very serious medical problems. *Necessary* is not really debatable.

Now let's tackle the ugly matter of the money.

I say "ugly" because nobody really likes talking about this. Most orthodontists are nervous about it. Parents are uncomfortable with it. If there is a financial obstacle to treatment, most people are reluctant to admit it, offer other excuses, and then can't be helped by the doctor. I think we have to trust each other. With me, this discussion is entirely confidential, in a "safe zone." Orthodontists are not Martians, by the way; we have kids, college tuitions that loom, and family budgets.

What Is a Reasonable Fee and Cost?

A complete treatment program, including braces, can cost anywhere from $4,000 to $10,000 or so. Most fall in between. Adjusted for inflation, these prices are actually *less than* braces decades ago, while the technology and quality has advanced. In costs it can prevent later, it's a bona fide bargain. TMJ treatments are expensive. Cosmetic dentistry work is expensive. Migraine headache drugs are expensive and have side effects.

For this investment, you will be getting the carefully selected, personalized solution to your child's irregularities and problems, prescribed using state-of-the-art digital technology along with the expertise of a specialist, and considerate, compassionate care from start to finish. Your investment includes a varying number of appointments plus the orthodontic appliance itself, after-care, and in my office, certain guarantees.

It's hard to really draw a fair comparison, but if you have any significant net worth, you can easily pay similar fees for the services of an attorney expert in estate planning. Most kitchen remodels cost considerably more. Where real expertise is involved and the stakes of getting it wrong are high, you can't escape professional level fees.

In this case, the $4,000 to $10,000 range is seen as perfectly reasonable by the overwhelming majority of parents that I talk to. Each year, we provide braces of one kind or another to countless patients. Even parents who shook their heads at the cost to start with tell me afterward that having witnessed everything we do to get the absolute best obtainable results, and seeing the outcome itself, they feel undercharged.

While it's never easy to part with such a sum, people do it every day for all sorts of less important things, and when they do often pay for something like their new designer handbag, golf vacation, or suite of living room furniture. They'll pay for it outright or with their favorite credit card (getting the reward points in the bargain). If you put the orthodontic treatment program including braces on a typical credit card at the interest in play as I write this, and you choose to make only the minimum required monthly payment, your monthly payments will be relatively small. Even tight budgets can accommodate this *when it is really important*. It's less than most families pay for their cable and streaming entertainment. For many, if they got all their Starbucks stops consolidated into one monthly bill, it would be more than this!

Health Spending Accounts (HSA) /Flex Spending Accounts (FSA)

The HSA allows you to set aside pre-tax dollars to be used for certain medical and health expenses for you or your family. They exist although restricted under the Affordable Care Act (Obamacare) as it stood in July of 2017. By the time you read this, the opportunity may have been expanded, as President Trump suggested. In any case, if you have accumulated money in an HSA, you can probably spend it on orthodontic treatment. If you don't have an HSA, you might want to start one. Information can be found online about existing or new accounts and their rules of use, at www.healthcare.gov.

Other kinds of FSAs are typically set up through your place of employment and similarly enable you to set aside pre-tax dollars for medical expenses. Sometimes, employers match contributions. Again, you can almost certainly tap funds from your FSA for your child's orthodontic care. Check with your employer about this.

If you have a tax accountant, you may want to consult with him about your HSA or FSA.

> *TIP:*   *How can you make the most out of your employer's*
> *flex-pay plan?*
>
> First, make sure you understand how it works. Second, set aside flex-spending dollars in advance of need, and if possible, make the maximum contributions. Many employers allow higher limits than you'd think without asking, as much as $2,500 to $5,000 per year. Be aware of "family status changes" allowed by your plan that may enable you to change the amount being moved pre-tax from your paychecks to your account anytime during the year rather than just once at the first of the year—so you could bump up the amount in months before the first orthodontic treatment. **IMPORTANT:** Be aware of the balance and the loss of unused funds. In most cases, if you do not use these funds, you lose them, year to year. You usually have three months after the end of the calendar year to submit claims for eligible expenses from the previous year.

Insurance

These days, there are as many different types of insurance plans as there are patients in my office. I can't possibly speak to your unique and personal insurance policy without seeing it first but, in general, my experience tells me that "most" insurance policies cover "some" of your orthodontic expenses.

I realize that answer sounds very vague, but here are a couple of variables you need to answer before an insurance agent can help you determine what, how long, and how many procedures fall under your insurance:

- The type of procedure (braces, Invisalign, etc.)
- The duration of the procedure (two months, six months, a year, etc.)
- The cause of the procedure (a patient presenting with pain, a parent's concern, traumatic injury or accident, congenital birth defect like cleft lip or palate etc.)
- The nature of the procedure (to correct pain/discomfort, cosmetic, etc.)

I can only partially answer this question, but talking to your insurance agent will help you get the right answers you need.

TIP: *Keep an insurance journal of every interaction with your carrier.*

Write down the date, time of call, name of the person you contacted, and the exact instructions or recommendations following the call.

Later, if your insurance company doesn't remember what they told you, you'll have it accurately written down. If they still don't remember, ask them to pull the recorded audio tape from your previous call, so that you can accurately "remind" them of exactly what they told you.

Loans

If you have equity in your home, the lowest-cost loan option may be a home equity line of credit or second mortgage. See your own bank, or check out RocketMortgage at rocket.quickenloans.com. As of this writing, mortgage interest is at record lows.

Obviously, a private loan from a family member can be the easiest option. A lot of preteens' and teens' important orthodontic care is financed at the Bank of Grandma and Grandpa.

If the other options are difficult or unavailable, we will set up a weekly, bimonthly, or monthly "paycheck payment plan" with a comfortable monthly payment.

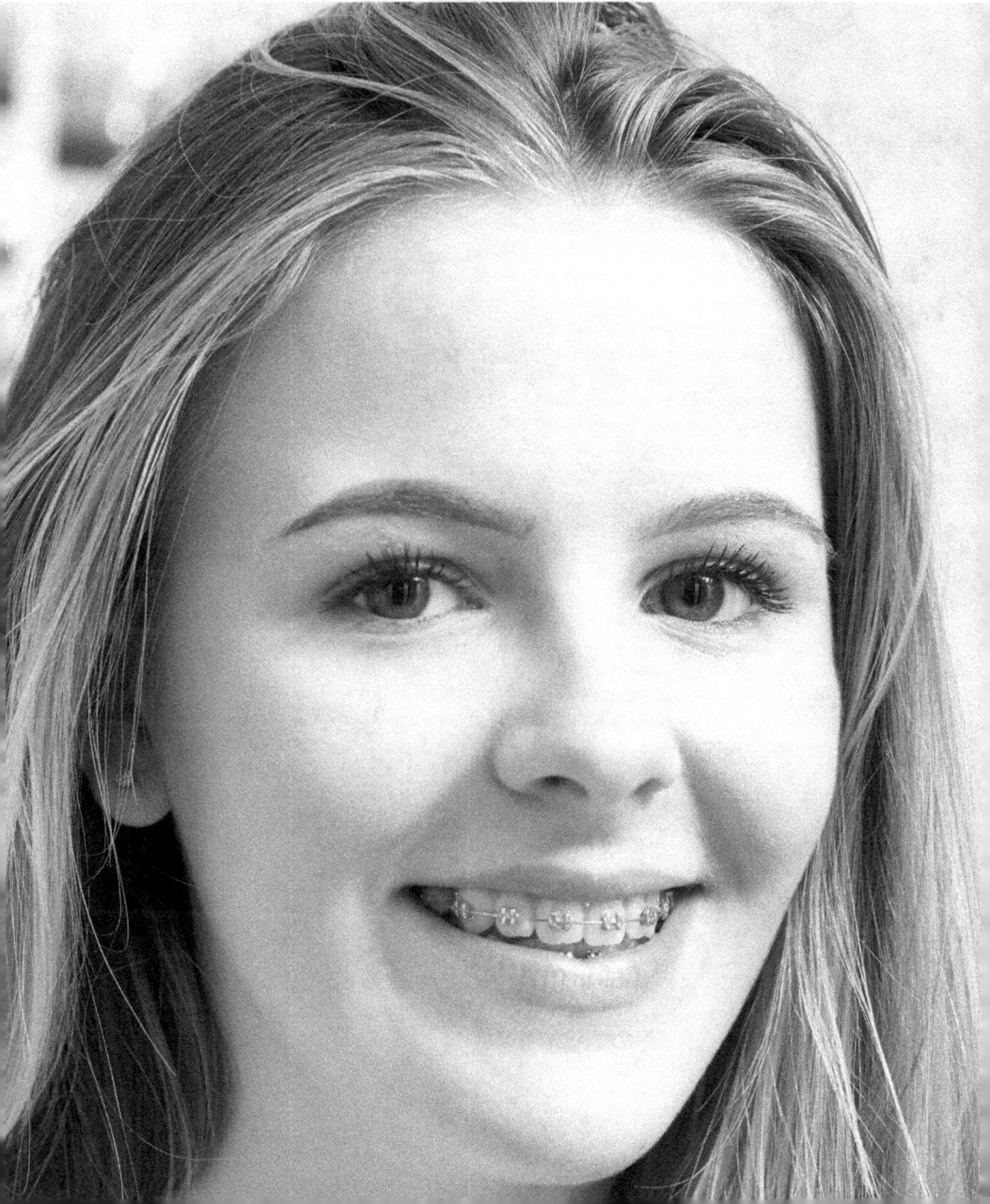

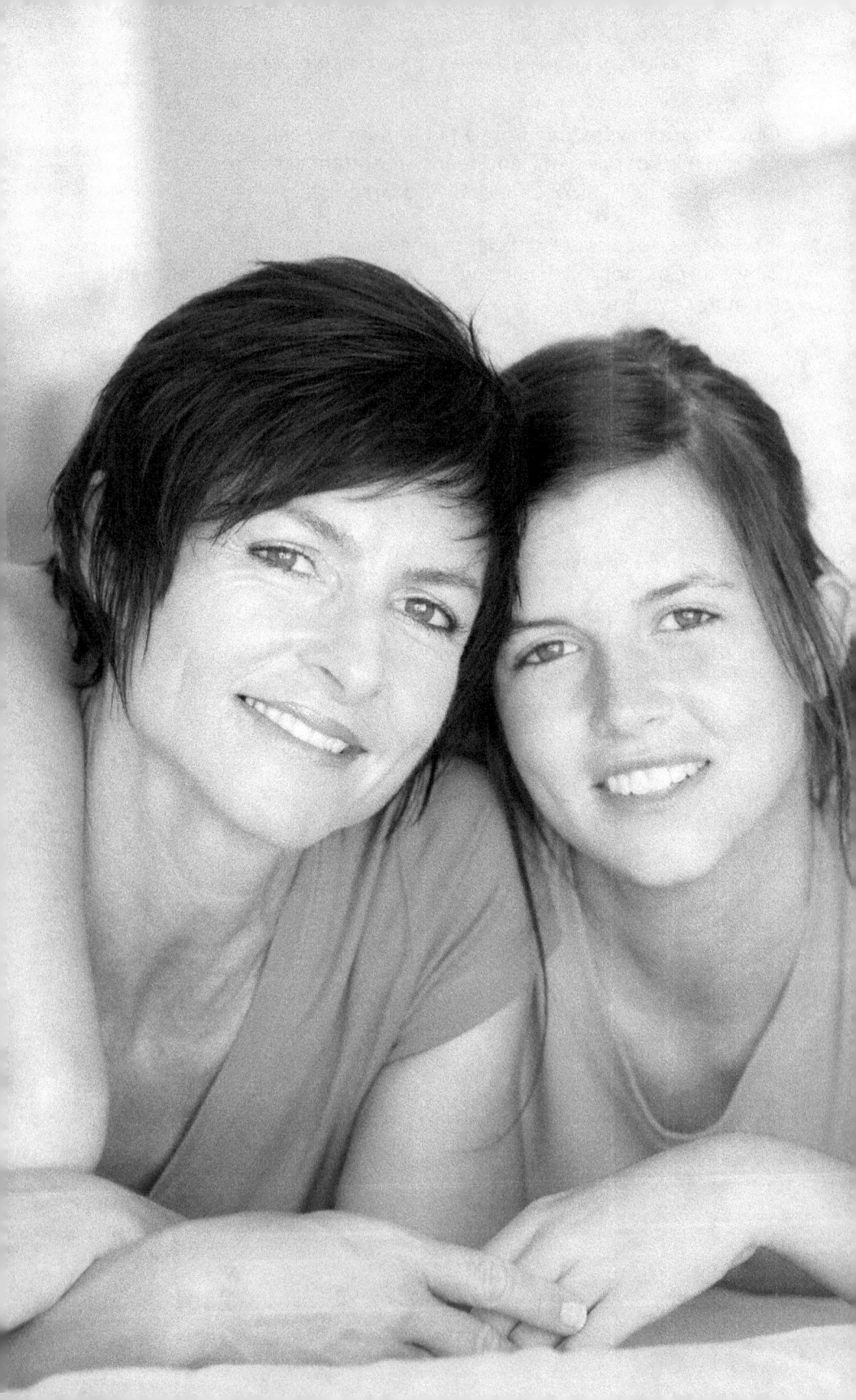

CHAPTER 9

What Are the Treatment Options?

If your child is ready for orthodontic care, one of the first discussions to have with your orthodontist is which procedure is right for him or her; there might be more options than you had ever imagined.

If you're like most people, you associate orthodontists with braces, but these days that is just one arm of what I or any orthodontist does. Here are some of the services most orthodontists will provide their patients with during the course of routine treatment:

- Metal, tie-free braces
- Invisalign clear removable aligners
- Clear braces
- Expanders to match jaw size and tooth size
- Habit appliances to eliminate thumb sucking
- Space maintainers
- Retainers to prevent crowding and shifting of teeth
- Functional appliances to help improve facial balance
- Early treatment and growth modification
- Customized appliances designed uniquely for each patient

While many of these services may seem self-explanatory to you, several will probably not. In the following pages, I will try to elaborate on several of them, including:

- Crossbite correction
- Metal braces
- Clear braces
- Invisalign

Crossbite Correction

As your child's teeth begin to grow in, there's a lot more at work than mere gum lines, tooth fairies, and molar size. How the jaw is shaped, when it develops, and even how "normally" it develops can all affect the placement and comfort of your child's teeth.

When the upper and lower teeth grow at different rates, or even when the lower jaw grows disproportionately with the upper jaw, something known as a "crossbite" can occur.

> *Your child might have a crossbite if, for instance, the lower jaw is out of line with the upper jaw (kind of like a box that won't close right because one of the hinges is bent).*

Or perhaps on the right side of your child's mouth, the lower teeth "stick out" a little farther than the top teeth, making the upper teeth on that side overlap in turn.

Or maybe your child's upper and lower jaws are out of alignment so instead of the top and bottom front teeth meeting "naturally" as they should, the front teeth fall somewhat behind the lower teeth. This would be the reverse of an overbite.

As you might imagine, any or all of these developments can lead to short- and long-term discomfort for your child.

How, When, and Why Crossbites Form

You might be amazed to find out how many ways a crossbite can form as your child grows and develops during his or her formative years. Heredity is one key to jaw growth, or alignment, as is the size of your child's developing jaw.

Another factor that can contribute to the development of a potential crossbite is if it takes your child too long to lose his or her baby teeth. In some extreme cases, in fact, if it takes too long for your child to lose his baby teeth, another set of teeth can grow in behind them, throwing the alignment off and contributing to a crossbite.

Believe it or not, something as basic as whether your child breathes through her nose or her mouth can also contribute to a crossbite. While most children breathe through their noses, some children develop a habit early on of breathing through their mouths instead.

In children who breathe through their noses while they're sleeping, the tongue naturally rests on the roof of the mouth, promoting natural and proper upper jaw growth. When young children breathe through their mouths, however, the tongue relocates from the roof of the mouth to the bottom, removing that extra support and potentially contributing to reduced upper jaw bone growth; this can create the crossbite we spoke of previously.

How Can I Spot a Crossbite?

Although it sounds severe, and even painful from the description provide earlier, the effects of a crossbite can take time to manifest themselves. Still, here are some of the telltale signs your child might be cultivating, or already suffering from, a crossbite:

- Snoring
- Difficulty breathing
- Chewing on one side of the mouth or the other
- Signs of an underbite
- If your child's chin seems "off center" or disproportionate

How, When, and Why to Correct a Crossbite

Where should you start looking for treatment if you're concerned about your child's jaw development after reading this section? If you suspect your child might have a crossbite, approach your family dentist about a recommendation for a specialist such as an orthodontist.

There are many possible treatments available for a crossbite, and your orthodontist can work with you closely to make the right and specific decisions for you and your child.

When should you start? I believe you know my standard answer when it comes to questions like this one: *as early as possible!* The same way an auto mechanic would tell you to take care of that oil leak, bulging tire, or faulty timing belt sooner rather than later, myself and my colleagues in orthodontics will always favor early treatment to later.

Crossbites are often closely linked with other orthodontic issues, such as teeth alignment, jaw size, and growth, so naturally, the sooner you address any or all of these issues, the better.

Finally, why should you address a crossbite? Crossbites can lead to pain, discomfort, and a lack of confidence as your child begins to feel insecure or even ostracized because of this very treatable, very normal series of jaw and teeth developments.

Not only can crossbites become physically uncomfortable if left untreated, but if the misalignment or root cause of the bite isn't fixed early in childhood, then the child's appearance and, ultimately, confidence could be affected as the crossbite becomes more pronounced in adolescence.

Metal Braces

The fact is, metal braces still have a valued place in the orthodontic world, and despite advances and breakthroughs of products like Invisalign and even clear braces, they aren't going extinct anytime soon! This is because metal braces are very strong and can withstand most types of treatment. Today's metal braces are smaller, sleeker, and more polished than ever before.

You may have heard of "speed braces." These are sometimes also referred to as "self-ligating brackets" or "tie-free braces." Self-ligating means that the brackets do not need the little o-shaped rubber bands (ligatures) or metal tie wires to hold the arch wire onto the bracket. Several companies have developed braces for holding the wires in place without ligatures.

By using self-ligation technology, the brackets allow the wire to slide back and forth. This advancement allows for fewer adjustments and fewer appointments. These types of braces do not need rubber bands to hold the arch wire in place. They use a "door" to secure the arch wire to the bracket. They're smaller than traditional metal and less food gets trapped around them when you eat.

Your orthodontist might use an advanced self-ligating bracket that does not require physical tightening of the wire to the braces. It's a twin bracket made of metal or clear ceramic and utilizes a special built-in clip. The pressure from specific types of arch wires activates the clip and delivers specific amounts of force to each tooth, resulting in fast, directed results.

Naturally, orthodontists are very excited about the hygiene benefits of these self-closing or tie-free metal braces. Patients are excited that their braces are small, smooth, and friction-free and straighten their teeth in fewer visits with less discomfort than braces with wires that are "tied-in."

Gold Braces

We now offer gold braces. The appearance is more subtle and my staff & patients love them! And as of this writing, we are the only office in the area providing this style of treatment.

Clear Braces

Ceramic braces are very strong and generally do not stain. Adults like to choose ceramic because they "blend in" with the teeth and are less noticeable than metal. These are the type of braces actor Tom Cruise had.

Adult Orthodontics

It's not uncommon for individuals who have undergone orthodontic treatment earlier in life to find their teeth have drifted out of alignment over the years. Most adults won't think twice about bleaching their teeth to roll back the effects of time. Yet few think about the role orthodontics can play.

Adults of all ages can enjoy the same cosmetic and health benefits of properly aligned teeth with appliances like the In-Ovation C system braces.

Improperly aligned teeth can do more than undermine your confidence. They can make proper cleaning and brushing more difficult, contribute to enamel loss and even set the stage for more significant problems down the road. Fortunately, discrete treatment can help keep you aligned with a healthy, happy lifestyle.

Clear Correct - Clear Aligners

Clear Correct is a widely advertised, well-known, and popular orthodontic product, and often, kids know about it and ask parents and doctors for it by name. For many, it's as good an option as any other and sometimes even the best option.

Clear Correct uses advanced, proprietary 3-D computer imaging technology to "map" the entire span of treatment, from the present teeth alignment to the desired positioning, alignment, and smile. Clear aligners are custom made and based on the 3-D imaging. Clear Correct has many features that have helped make it such a popular choice. The aligners are removable, even before a snack or meal as well as for general hygiene. There are no metal brackets or wires. Office visits for adjustments throughout the treatment program are fast, easy and painless. The thermoplastic aligners are virtually invisible.

At the start, we determine whether you or your child is a good candidate for the Clear Correct approach, or if they would be better served with different braces. You have to rely on *somebody* to tell you. I promise you, there are kids who've been hurried to Clear Correct who were not good candidates for it.

Trustworthy, Objective Advice

Bluffton Orthodontics is *not* "in the pocket of" or obligated to any of these providers of different braces products and technologies. We select and recommend what we believe is the most appropriate and beneficial choice for your child. We are happy to discuss the pros and cons of different ones, if your child has heart set on, say, Invisalign, because that's what a friend has, or based on information you've obtained.

Candidly, these manufacturers vary in price to the orthodontist (or dentist) based on volume purchase benchmarks, incentivizing concentration of as much use as possible to one product. Awards are given out to the highest volume buyers and users. It's borderline unseemly. It introduces temptation into the diagnostic and prescriptive process, and I never let us bow to such incentives and temptations. The number-one rule here is: what is absolutely best for the patient?

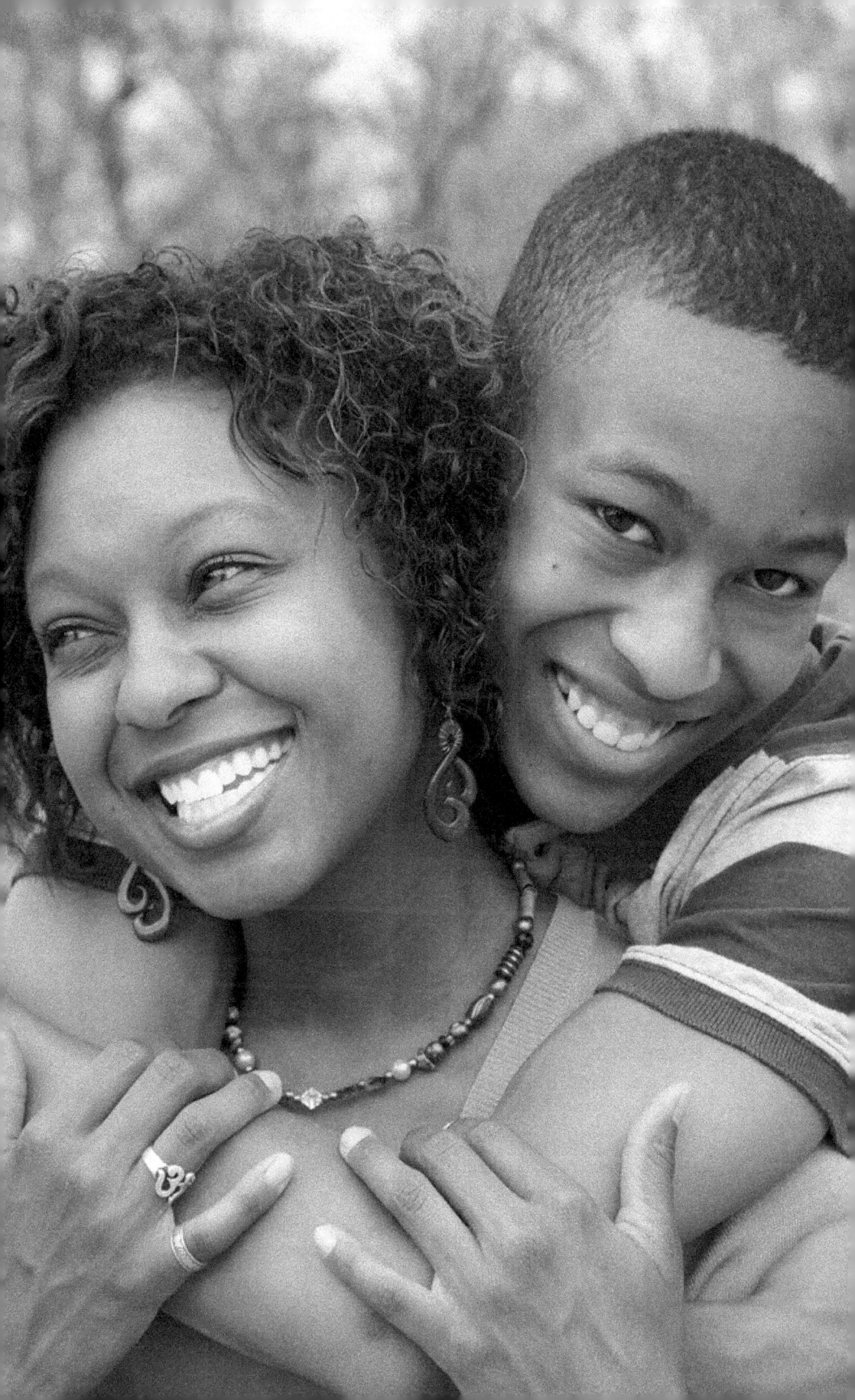

CHAPTER 10

How Difficult is Living with Braces?

Remember, this *isn't* 1982. Or 1992. Today's braces aren't anything like yours if you had them decades ago. Today's orthodontic care is far more advanced, more sophisticated, and more patient-centered than any prior generation has experienced. If you had traditional metal braces twenty years or so ago, you experienced medieval torture. The dungeon is gone too, replaced by ultra-modern, patient comfort friendly offices. Out of the dark, into the light!

Living with braces is not going to be anywhere near as difficult as you might imagine.

Let's look at a few specific concerns.

Brushing and Hygiene

Modern braces, whether they're metal, flexible, or "invisible," are all actually made to fit the individual and facilitate easy, painless, thorough brushing. This means your child brushes pretty much the same as he would if he didn't have braces.

Here are some simple tips you can share with your child for the best results when brushing with braces on:

- Brush your teeth with a soft nylon toothbrush after you eat and before bed*
- Brush, rinse, and look; if you find any areas that are not clean, brush them again.
- Brush your gums as you brush your teeth (massage and stimulate).
- Take extra care in the area between the gums and the braces, because food caught and left there can cause swollen gums, cavities, discomfort, and permanent teeth stains.
- If no toothpaste is available, brush without.
- If you are unable to brush, rinse your mouth vigorously with water.
- Replace your old toothbrush when it gets worn out.
- It's absolutely essential you continue regular visits to your family dentist for checkups and cleanings throughout your orthodontic treatment!

---

* At my office, you'll be provided with a home kit including the best toothbrush, toothpaste, and rinse.

Depending on the age of your child, you, the parent, may need to supervise the first few brushings with the braces in place. You should not have a whining, resistant, difficult child on your hands because of any of this. It should be painless, simple, and routine.

Forbidden Foods Your Child Must Avoid

After your child's orthodontic appliance/braces have been placed, the teeth are usually "tender" and sensitive for as few as three to as many as ten days: a *short* time. During these few days, softer foods are recommended: soups, macaroni, spaghetti, eggs, fish, Jell-O, yogurt. As needed, Tylenol or Advil are adequate in relieving any discomfort, taken an hour or so before eating.* Warm saltwater rinses can be helpful. We also provide a "soft white wax," a safe topical that eases gum discomfort.

For the entire duration of the braces being in place, I'd advise you to stay away from hard and sticky foods that can damage braces and may lengthen the time they have to be worn or even require extra office visits. Sugar-rich foods can make hygiene harder and cause calculus build-up and cavities. You're probably already monitoring and limiting your child's intake of such foods, so there's really nothing new under the sun here. But, for the record, here are the "featured items" that should be avoided during orthodontic treatment and wearing of braces:

1. **Rock-hard foods:** Ice (don't chew ice!), nuts, popcorn (has hard kernels inside), peanut brittle, rock candy, whole apples and carrots (unless cut into bite sized pieces), corn on the cob, hard pretzels, hard rolls, hard taco shells.

2. **Extra-sticky foods:** Jolly Ranchers or Starbursts or similar candies, bubble gum, taffy, and sticky Cinnabon rolls.

3. **Very chewy foods:** Pizza crust, beef jerky, gummy bears. Note: no chewing on pencils or pens.

4. **Super-sugary foods and drinks:** Limit sodas and sugary foods.

We will speak about this with your son or daughter and give them a printed list, but you will have to reinforce, monitor, and provide some substitute foods to prevent mutiny or months of sulking. Most kids get it, though. When they understand how short or long the number of weeks of wearing braces will turn out to be, how comfortable or uncomfortable wearing them and hygiene while wearing them is, and how successful the outcome will be is linked to their staying away from the short list of harmful foods, they are pretty responsible about it. Most parents who are initially really worried about this tell us later it wasn't the horror show they'd imagined.

Emergencies, Injuries, Travel, and Time Away from Home

Many "emergencies" actually aren't and can be easily and safely remedied at home. You are provided with a "What to Do in Case of the 5 Common Emergencies" printed card, and you can always access the same information at our web site, 24/7/365.

Common emergencies include the breaking of some part of the braces, eating something particularly damaging—even a McDonalds bun full of sesame seeds might feel like an emergency, or, early, a feeling of discomfort that worries something serious might be wrong. These are the sort of things addressed in the "What to Do" instructions.

If you do run up against an emergency that isn't easily managed with these instructions or can't wait for regular office hours, we have a special phone number to call that routes to a knowledgeable staff member directly or with return call within sixty minutes or less.

If your family or son or daughter are away from home and say, they chomp down on a piece of toffee and break a piece of their braces, there is *always* a remedy. You are *not* going to cut your vacation short and rush to the airport! Again, often a remedy you do by our instructions can meet the urgent need until everybody gets back home.

Sports

Speaking of injuries, the question of sports versus braces worries kids and parents alike. These days, kids are *very* active in organized and school sports, some starting one as another's season is ending. You know this; you are coordinating the schedules and working as their unpaid chauffeur.

Good news: for every sport and every level of play, there is either an inexpensive off-the-shelf mouth guard or a slightly costlier, custom-fit mouth guard to provide an extra, suitable level of dental protection and to protect the braces themselves. In some sports, additional face masks or other equipment normally treated as an option can be added and used during the time period of the orthodontic treatment.

We have thought this through! For example, research reported in Clinics in Sports Medicine, from the Department of Neurology at Boston University School of Medicine examined uses of different kinds of mouth guards and the rate of sports-related concussions. There was no significant difference in concussion risks found tied to different types of mouth guards.

By the way, there are collegiate and pro athletes, even NFL players, getting orthodontic treatment and even wearing braces. If they can, your child can! You do *not* need the drama of stopping your child from playing the sports they're committed to because of their orthodontic treatment. Oh, and we even guarantee your office visits will not cause you to miss work or business responsibilities, nor cause your child to miss school or organized sports.

See, this *isn't* going to be difficult!

Tips for Helping Your Child Adjust to a Life with Braces

- **All the cool kids are doing it (or soon will be):** Braces are a very popular appliance during the middle school and high school years. Rather than focus on how he or she feels wearing braces, encourage your child to begin actively looking for other kids who are wearing braces. Chances are, they'll find lots more than they ever imagined!

- **Even famous people do it:** Gwen Stefani. Prince Harry. Drew Barrymore. Tom Cruise. Dakota Fanning. Danny Glover. The list of famous people who've worn braces—many of them as adults—could fill half this book. Share with your child how even the most famous people in the spotlight sometimes need a little help through braces.

- **Be prepared:** Finally, create a "master list" of things your child likes to do: things that make him feel special, confident, brave, calm, relaxed, or excited. If you notice him feeling down, consult your list and make plans to do something special in the near future to boost his confidence level back to where you know it belongs!

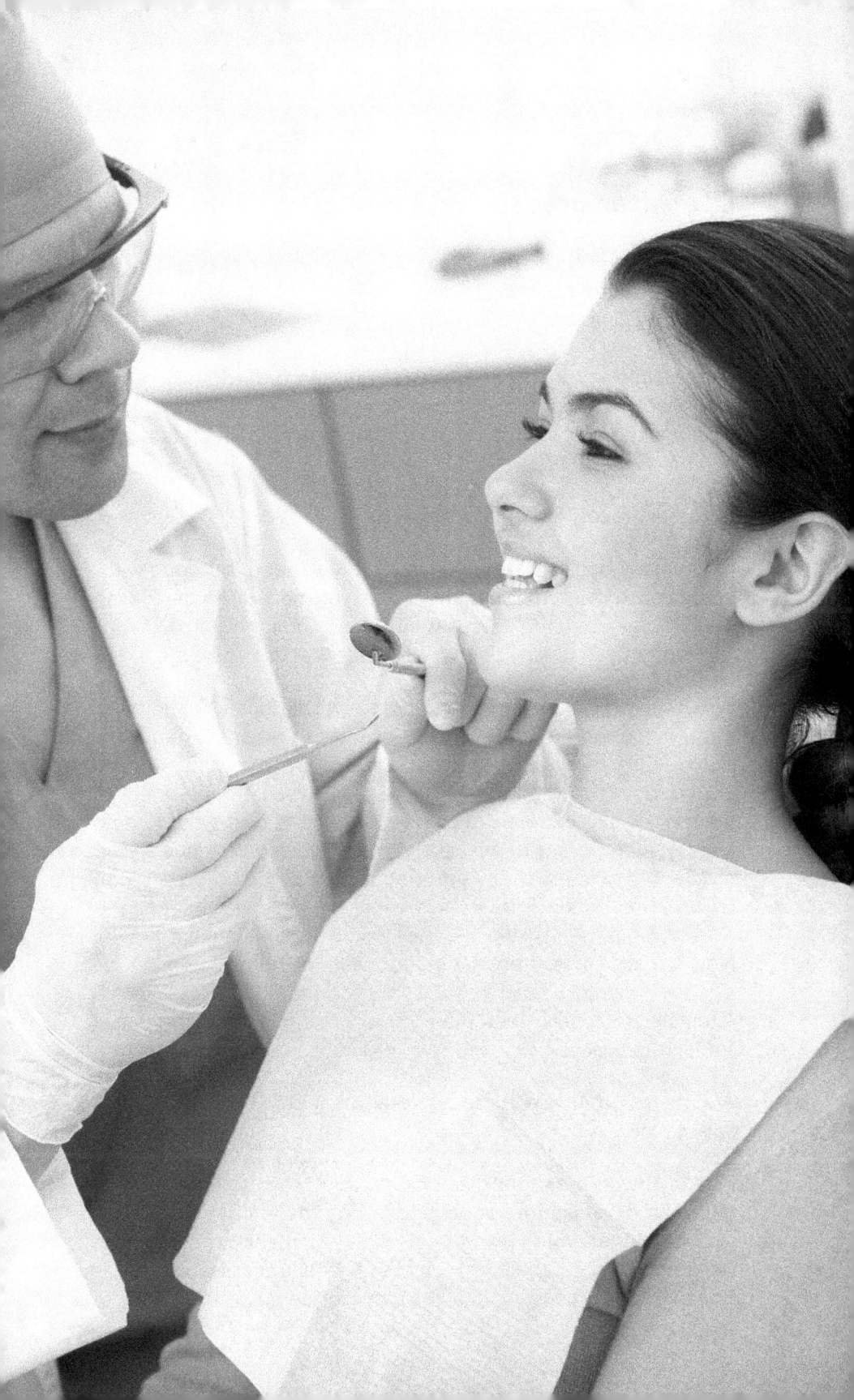

CHAPTER 11

Life After Braces: Retainers

So, your child's braces are off and they're ready to live a life full of confidence and good oral health. They may think, *I'm free! I'm free!* Well, not quite yet.

The selection of the right braces, the expert orthodontist, and the compliant wearing of the braces gets us about three-fourths of the way to where we want to be: a well-aligned, as-perfect-as-possible, healthy smile for life.

But after braces, there are retainers.

While many patients are understandably eager to be done with braces once they come off, the fact is, retainers do as much work— if not more—than the braces themselves. Straight teeth in proper alignment have to stay that way, and for that, retainers are a big help.

When the braces are removed, teeth can still shift if not helped through a period of adjustment, to settle in. Retainers gently but purposefully remind the teeth to stay straight during this adjustment period. It's advised that nearly all patients who've gone through the time, work, and expense of braces will want to use fixed or removable retainers for months or years or even for life and continue to schedule regular orthodontic check-ups. Some dentists doing braces won't tell you this, but I will. Years ago, clinicians believed that once teeth were straightened by braces, they would simply stay that way forever. New science says otherwise. In fact, teeth position shifting as we age is to be expected. Teeth naturally shift to the middle and crowd. So, retainers are actually extremely important in maintaining the new smile from braces.

Any claims otherwise, by some "brand" of braces or any doctor, are flat-out false.

In post-braces monitoring and check-ups, I tend to decide on the best kind of retainer for your child before the removal of the braces. Growth of the jaw following treatment (yes, the jaw is still growing in adolescents, to age eighteen or so), stabilizing of the gums and bone tissues, pressures from lips and tongue, and other factors tell me what type of retainer should be worn and for how long. Retainers are made out of rubber, plastic, and sometimes, still metal. They are custom made and fit, as part of the complete orthodontic treatment. However, after the initial orthodontic exam, at the same time the best braces are being selected, it's usually possible, with a good degree of certainty, to predict the type of retainer(s) your child is going to need, and I'm happy to share that information with you at that time.

Some retainers are invisible or nearly invisible. There are clear plastic retainers. A *fixed* retainer is typically placed on the inside/back surfaces of the lower front teeth. A fixed retainer may be used until lower jaw growth is complete and then no longer needed. When your child hears "retainer" he will most likely picture a *removable* retainer. These make hygiene easy, are easily removed and cleaned daily and can be removed for a sports activity.

There are even "fashion retainers" now—popular with kids of different ages—in school colors, and some even with pictures on them! In my office, patients using different kinds of retainers also receive clear, flexible plastic retainers as a back-up in case of damage to the main retainer or for occasional social functions where the preteen or teen "just can't be caught dead with a retainer in her mouth."

This is an important part of braces aftercare and part of the complete orthodontic treatment program personalized for your child.

Call us at 843-815-2521 or go to www.blufftonorthodontics.com
to schedule your own Customized Smile Analysis.

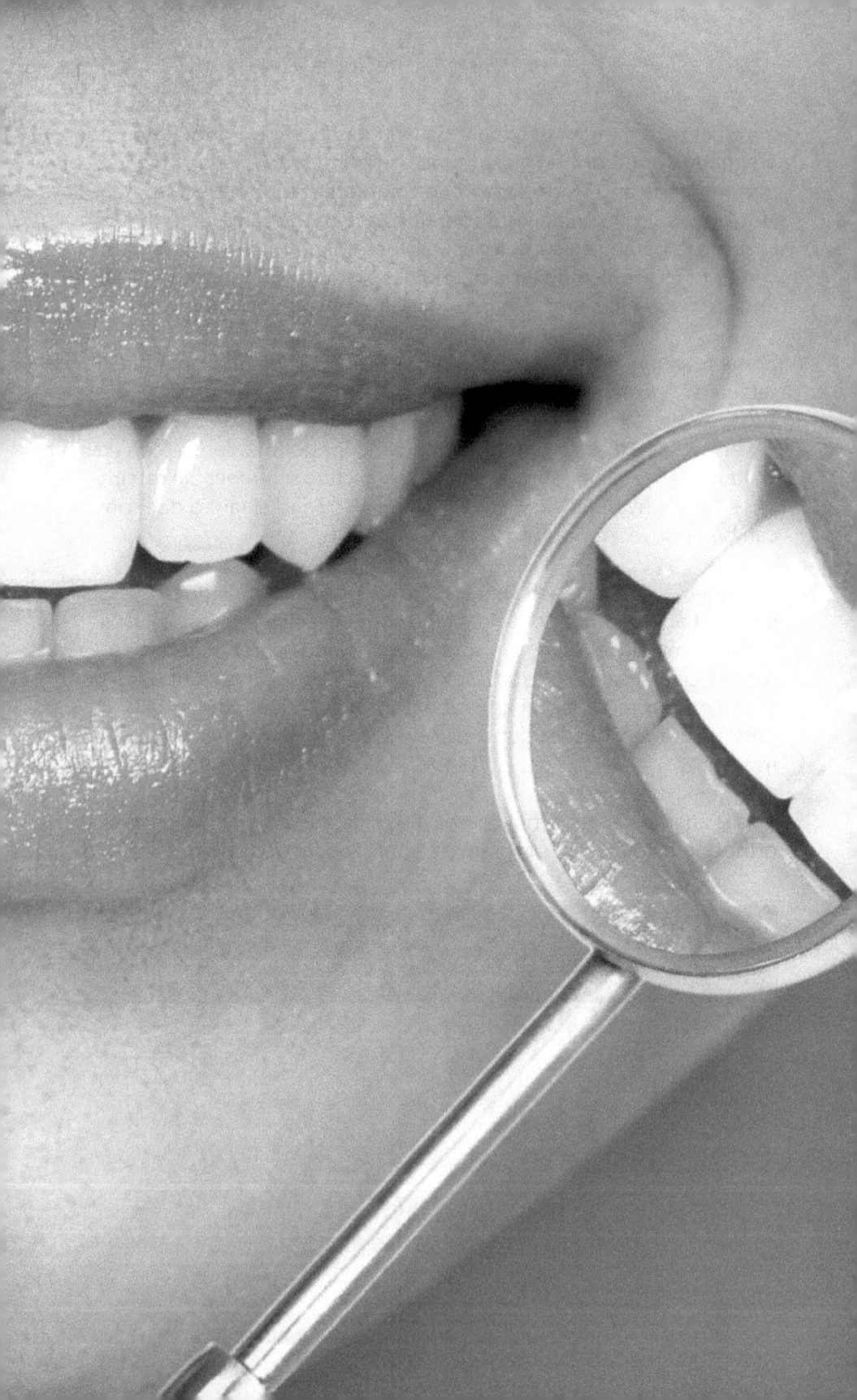

CHAPTER 12

Life After Braces: Wisdom Teeth

I hear many concerns from our patients receiving orthodontic treatment. It's not uncommon to hear things like *"How long do you have to wear my braces?"*, *"Will they hurt?"*, *"Will my wisdom teeth affect anything?"*

Wait, did you say wisdom teeth?

I did! Wisdom teeth might not be on your radar, but a lot of our patients are very concerned about how their wisdom teeth can affect the outcome of their newly straighten smile. Some patients start to worry when they see their wisdom teeth beginning to emerge, thinking that they will mess up all the treatment they just underwent or are still finishing up.

Is this something to worry about? Can teeth exert enough pressure to move the teeth that are around them? Your worries are justifiable, but we've got you covered! Let's look at how wisdom teeth can affect orthodontic treatment!

First of all, what are wisdom teeth?

Wisdom teeth are the third set of adult molars. They usually make an appearance between the ages of 17–21. Some have theirs come in completely, while others' only come in partially. There are even a few people whose wisdom teeth don't come in at all!

Are wisdom teeth going to affect your smile?

Around the time that wisdom teeth start to come in, many patients will notice a "relapse" in their teeth positions. Are wisdom teeth really the reason for this shift?

You might find this surprising, but studies show that wisdom teeth are not to blame! Most people assume that because wisdom teeth grow in sideways that they must exert quite a bit of pressure on the teeth next to them and cause teeth to shift. However, research has shown that wisdom teeth do not exert the amount of pressure needed to move the teeth in front of them to cause the shift. Researchers place sensors between patients' teeth and observed the pressure on them, both with and without wisdom teeth present. There was no visible difference. So, if wisdom teeth don't cause your teeth to shift in your late teens and early twenties, then what does?

The answer no one wants to hear: We get older!

It's perfectly normal for our teeth to start to change as we get older. They might begin to overlap as part of a natural drifting that occurs, moving teeth forward slightly. As they begin to overlap, the upper teeth will sometimes press the lower teeth inward toward the tongue. Also, around this time of life, the jaw does undergo a growth spurt which can also move teeth into some less than desirable positions.

So, if you've ever wondered why we encourage you to wear your retainer so much, now you know! Wearing your retainer is the best defense to help your teeth stay as straight as they were when you finished your orthodontic treatment!

A Little Wisdom about Wisdom Teeth

Even though wisdom teeth might not affect your newly straighten smile, there are a few oral health concerns you might want to keep in mind if yours are growing in. These concerns can cause some oral health issues:

- If wisdom teeth only emerge partially, a flap of skin can potential form that partially covers the tooth and has a bad habit of trapping food. This can cause gum infection and tooth decay if it is not taken care of.

- Some people don't have enough room in their mouth for their wisdom teeth to fully emerge. When this happens, they often end up impacted. This means that they can break through the surface and get stuck in your jaws and gums, which can cause some discomfort.

- If the they do become impacted, painful cysts can sometimes form on the gums. These cysts can sometimes cause infection and decay to the tooth roots surrounding them.

- Wisdom teeth often emerge sideways or at an awkward angle. If this happens they can rub against the inside of the cheeks and cause discomfort.

One of the biggest concerns we see with wisdom teeth is that many patients don't have enough room for them to come in comfortably. Even if there is enough room for their wisdom teeth, the back of the mouth is usually so crowded that brushing and flossing them proves to be very difficult. This is one of the leading causes of tooth decay and gum infection in the back of the mouth.

Don't skip the retainer!

If you have already had orthodontic treatment, the best thing that you can do to keep your teeth from shifting is wearing your retainer consistently. If you notice your wisdom teeth starting to emerge, give us a call to avoid any of the potential problems that come with impacted or partially emerged wisdom teeth. You should also continue to schedule regular appointments with us or your dentist even after your orthodontic treatment is finished.

To wrap it all up...

Thankfully, problems with overcrowding can be diagnosed long before wisdom teeth ever make their appearance. Once they get close enough to the surface, they can be easily extracted to prevent further complications.

If you're worried about your wisdom teeth coming in during your orthodontic treatment, don't be! Wisdom teeth can't easily be removed while also having braces, so you don't have to worry about how they will affect your treatment. Your treatment will continue uninterrupted!

Not every person has to have their wisdom teeth removed. If you're one of the lucky ones not experiencing problems with yours, then there is no need to have them extracted.

Once again, we cannot emphasize enough how important it is to continuously wear your retainer after finishing up your orthodontic treatment. It's the only sure-fire way to keep your teeth looking as straight as they did when you finished your treatment. If you start to notice that yours is feeling tighter than normal or that there's a bit of pressure in the back of your mouth, schedule a visit with us so that we can determine whether or not it is your wisdom teeth coming in.

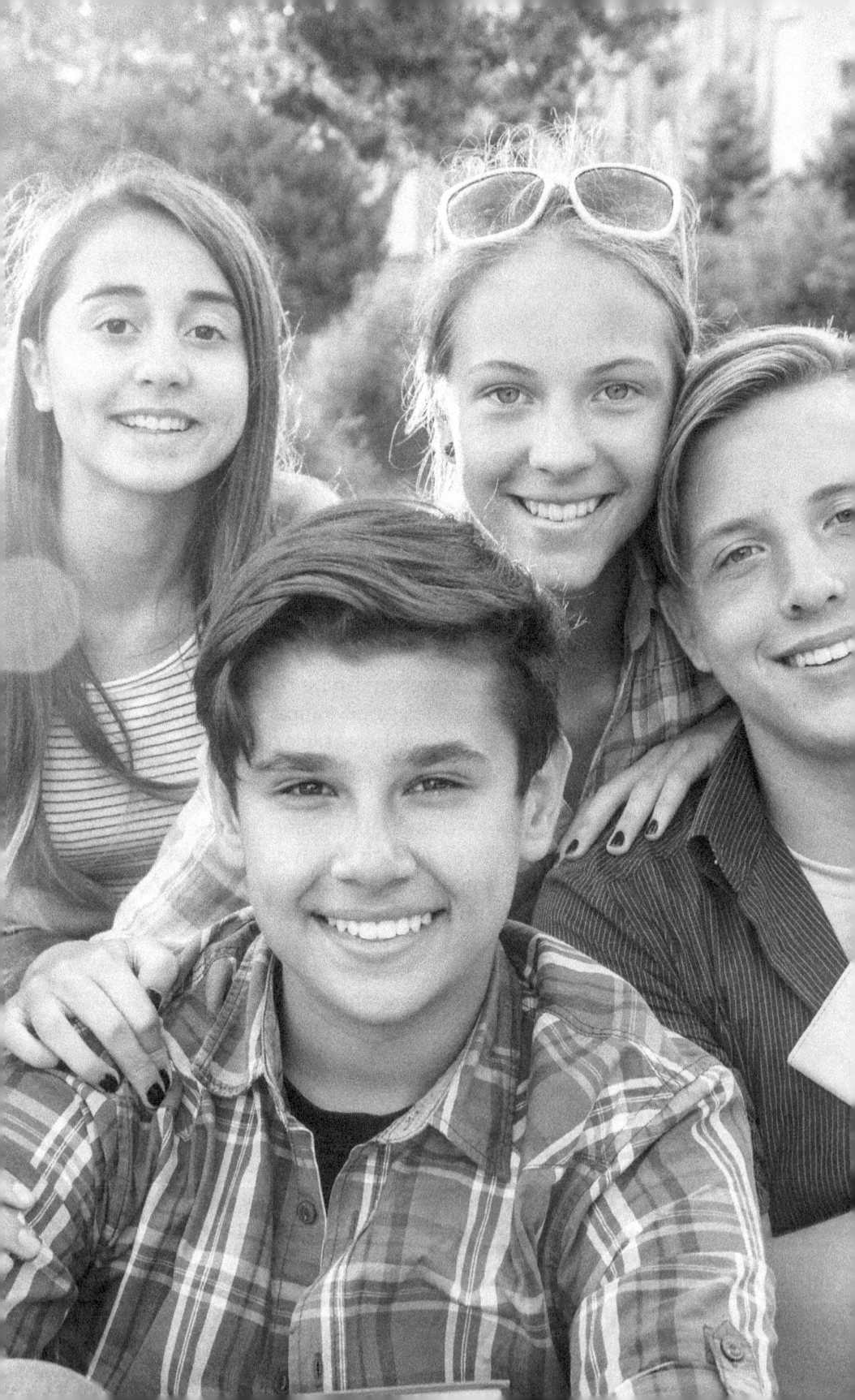

CHAPTER 13

Let's Celebrate!

Having to wear braces can last for six months to two years or more in certain cases. During the time your child has them, they may have moved from child to preteen or preteen to teen, at times felt embarrassed by having them, and possibly missed out on some things. They probably gave up favorite foods and snacks. They at least had to be super-conscious of what they ate and didn't eat. It's been a long time since they could sink their teeth into an apple!

You endured whatever complaining there was. You traded time to the office visits. You dealt with the "uh-oh!" and "now what did you do?" emergencies if there were any. And, of course, you paid the bill.

We like to see our patients celebrate getting their braces off. There are so many ways your child can celebrate, everything from writing a journal about their experience to recording a video that shares their experience and shows their new look.

Here are a few options your child may want to consider:

- **Throw a party.** Throwing a "braces are off" party is a great way to celebrate. They can invite their friends over, put out the foods that they've been longing for, and they can enjoy showing off those new straight teeth. His friends will love being able to take part in the celebration.

- **Plan a photo shoot.** Your child deserves to show the world his new beautiful smile! Plan a photo shoot, so he can be one-on-one with a photographer and put his best smile forward. He'll get some great shots and can show all his friends on social media his new look.

- **Chew some gum.** Your child might have wanted to have gum for the longest time. Although it's not the best habit, she can take an afternoon to chew some gum and feel guilt and worry free. Chew to your heart's content!

- **Go caramel.** Now is the time your child can sink his teeth into something like a caramel apple. No more avoiding the caramel and cutting the apple into bite-sized pieces. Nope, he can actually eat a full caramel apple, right off the stick! He can get one at the mall or a carnival or even make them himself. Either way, he'll love being able to bite into that sticky, gooey sweetness worry free!

- **Picnic in the park.** Weather permitting, a picnic in the park will make for a fun celebration. Take some of your child's favorite outdoor games, invite the friends, and have a cooler filled with icy drinks. On the grill, you can plan for things like corn on the cob that your child had to largely avoid while having her braces. It will make for a memorable afternoon.

- **Have a potluck dinner.** Have your child's friends and family each bring a dish people with braces have to take precaution with. This will give them the chance to learn a little more about what you went through, and it'll be fun to see what options they come up with. Ask each of the guests to write down a comment about your child with or without her braces. Your potluck will be filled with interesting dishes, laughs, and a good time.

- **Relax.** What could be better than spending a couple of hours being pampered, or perhaps a round of golf or fishing out on the lake? Not much! Take your child out—celebrate them making it through their treatment. They'll walk out feeling and looking great.

Doing some of these things, such as chewing gum, may still not be good for your child's teeth or their body overall. But doing it on a special occasion, and not making a habit out of it, won't cause any harm.

Of course, nobody can celebrate unless we *started*. There really is no time like the present.

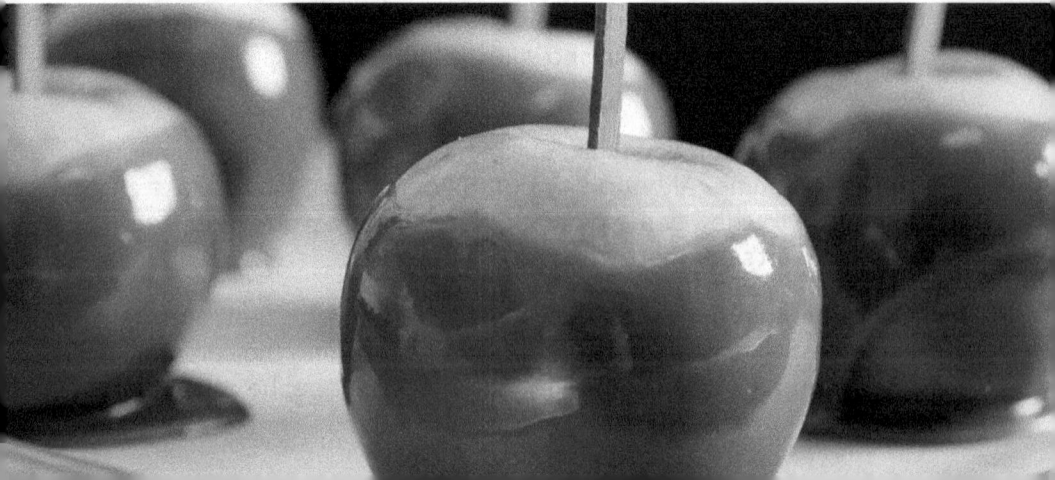

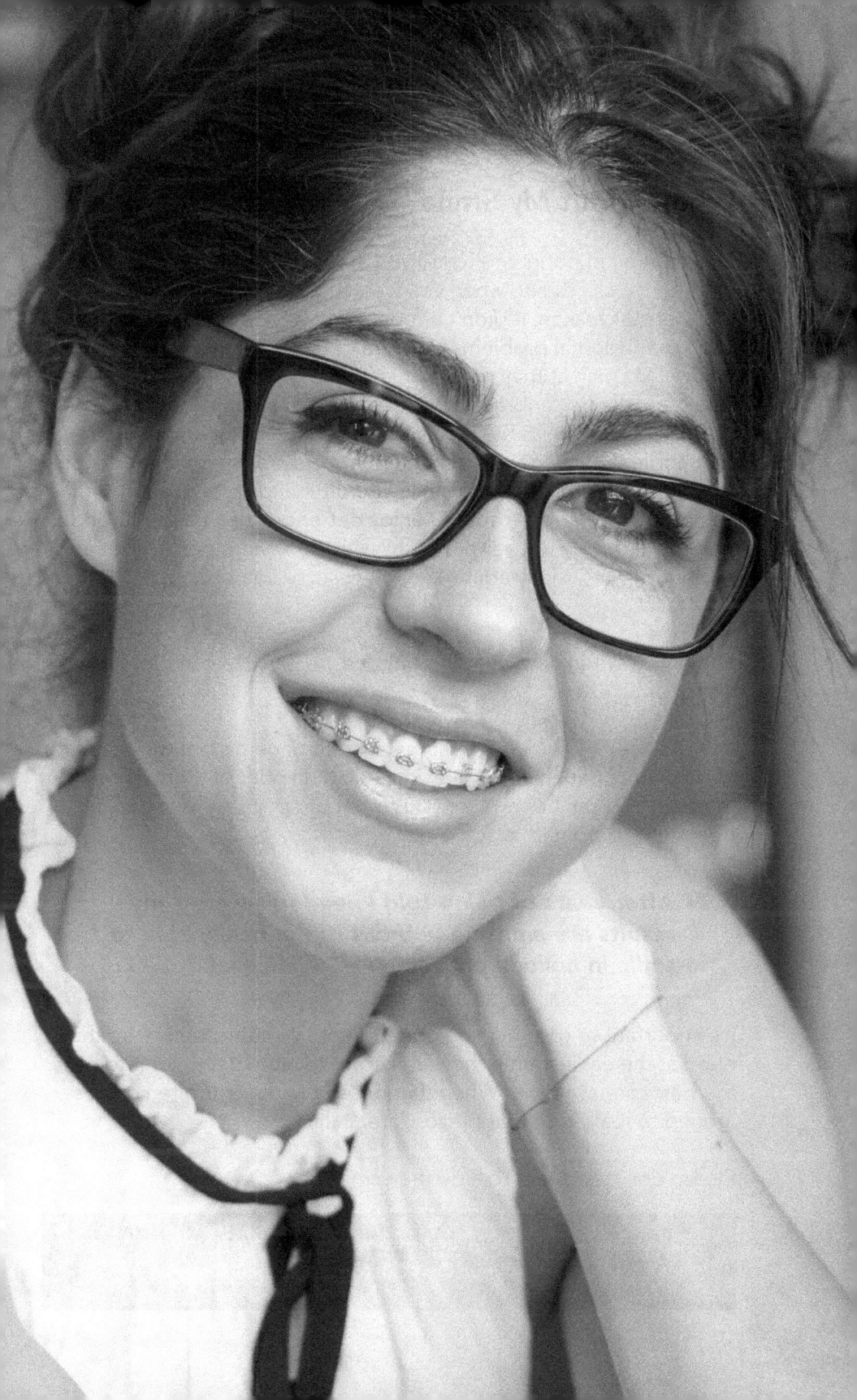

CHAPTER 14

What About My Smile?

Mom, Dad, I'm *not* going to kid you: if braces and/or orthodontic treatment was advised when you were eight or ten or twelve and, for whatever reason, it didn't happen, and you now have misaligned teeth, periodontal problems because of them, a smile you often hide, or jaw/TMJ pain, it may not be an easy fix. It may *not* even be fixable with orthodontics or braces. But often, to the surprise of adults, braces including invisible braces can do a significant amount of good for people thirty, forty, or even fifty years old. You may still be able to go from an embarrassing smile you often hide to a beautiful smile you love. You'll also be able to enjoy better oral health, gently and gradually over six to twelve months without having teeth pulled and without surgery. Many adults see ten years of age disappear from their faces.

The only way to know what the options are is with a complete, expert orthodontic exam.

At my office, we do not actively seek adult patients, but we treat a lot of parents of patients, just like you, and a number of them come from referrals. You can arrange for your exam by speaking to any of the treatment coordinators at the office.

> **❚❚ After years of being told I needed surgery, my results are amazing without it. I'm finally able to smile in holiday photos. ❚❚   — Michael R.**

It's important to get your son or daughter the orthodontic care they need at the earliest time they are known to need it and for it to be the best care available. When that doesn't happen, it often comes around to really bite that person later in life!

Please don't ask them to hide their smile!

Call us at 843-815-2521 or go to www.blufftonorthodontics.com to schedule your own Customized Smile Analysis.

FAQS

Here is a handy resource guide of frequently asked questions and orthodontic terminology, many of which are answered throughout the book.

What might happen if your child's mouth doesn't quite "fit"?
The fact is, the sooner you straighten your child's smile, the faster it will develop as it should: straight, clean, and healthy!

Who are some famous faces who've worn braces?
Gwen Stefani. Prince Harry. Drew Barrymore. Tom Cruise. Dakota Fanning. Danny Glover.

Will I be able to afford my child's braces?
Not only are most orthodontic procedures cheaper than ever, but insurance, payment plans, and a variety of other financing options make braces more affordable than they've ever been.

How much school will my child miss because of braces?
Not much, actually. After initial visits and, barring the actual procedure itself, most visits and/or adjustments are routine and can take anywhere from 15 to 45 minutes.

Is it really such a big deal if my child has crooked teeth?
Unfortunately, yes. Eroding, crooked, or unaligned smiles can take time to happen, but the time to act is now. Orthodontic irregularities don't just heal on their own or "go away" if you ignore them.

What are some of the warning signs that my child might need to go to the orthodontist?
There are many, but here are a few of the most common: early or late loss of teeth, protruding teeth, grinding or clenching of teeth, and speech difficulty.

What kind of "side effects" are caused by crooked teeth?

Some of the more frequent ones I see include headaches, toothaches, mouth breathing, chipped or worn down teeth, snoring, and drooling.

What makes an orthodontist more qualified than a dentist?

Orthodontists are dental specialists who have completed two to three years of additional education beyond dental school to learn the proper way to align teeth and jaws.

Why should I choose a specialist for my child's orthodontic care?

Unique treatment requirements and otherwise difficult bite problems are common, everyday scenarios for your orthodontist. In the interest of receiving the most efficient and effective orthodontic treatment possible, choose an orthodontic specialist.

How do I know if my doctor is an orthodontist?

Only orthodontists can belong to the American Association of Orthodontists (AAO).

What is a treatment coordinator?

During your initial consultation(s), you will usually be assigned a patient contact person—we call this person a "treatment coordinator" in our office—with whom to schedule appointments, confer with rescheduling and, of course, answer any and all questions you may have.

Why are follow-up visits important?

These are wonderful opportunities to either a.) ask questions you may have missed the first time or b.) get further details from your orthodontist him- or herself.

Why is early treatment so important?

Age seven is the earliest time your orthodontist can determine future jaw and tooth alignment. That's because, at the age of seven, your child's upper and lower permanent front teeth are developing. These teeth set the stage for future jaw position and serious problems can develop if they come into the wrong position.

What if I don't believe in early orthodontics?

Well, you're entitled to your opinion, but this is like saying you don't believe in the sun. You can hide from it, pretend it's not there, or refuse to acknowledge it, but the simple fact remains. If you're not aware of the potential risks, you can get burnt.

Will my child actually need braces at seven?

Probably not. While I inform parents their child needs an initial exam at age seven, I also mention that most children will not need braces until eleven to thirteen years of age.

What is a crossbite?

When the upper and lower teeth grow at different rates, or even when the lower jaw grows disproportionately with the upper jaw, something known as a "crossbite" can occur.

Where should I start to look for treatment if I'm concerned about my child's jaw development?

If you suspect your child might have a crossbite or other issues, approach your family dentist and ask about orthodontics.

Why should I address a crossbite?

Crossbites can lead to pain, discomfort, and lack of confidence as your child begins to feel insecure or even ostracized because of this very treatable, very normal series of jaw and teeth developments.

What is Clear Aligner Treatment?

Clear Aligner systems are the virtually invisible way to straighten your teeth and achieve the dazzling smile you've always dreamed of. Using advanced 3-D computer-imaging technology, Clear Correct depicts your complete treatment plan, from the initial position of your teeth to the final desired position.

Why are metal braces still so popular?

Metal braces are very strong and can withstand most types of treatment. Today's metal braces are smaller, sleeker, and more polished than ever before.

Are so-called "clear braces" effective?

Ceramic braces are very strong and generally do not stain. Adults like to choose ceramic braces because they "blend in" with the teeth and are less noticeable than metal. These are the types of braces actor Tom Cruise had.

What are some of my payment options in addition to insurance?

One way many patients pay for their procedures is by utilizing the benefits of what is known as "flex spending," where their employer matches their spending commitment.

What if my child has a "braces emergency" before or after office hours?

If you are experiencing an orthodontic emergency that can't wait for regular office hours, most orthodontic offices have a special number to call, either before, during, or after business hours. If this information isn't given to you readily, ask how your doctor's office handles emergencies.

Can a salt water rinse help deal with irritation caused by braces?

Absolutely; warm saltwater rinses soothe the cheek lining, which can get aggravated by your child's braces.

How do I make a salt water rinse?

To make a salt water rinse, mix ½ teaspoon of table salt in one cup of warm water. Stir until the salt is completely dissolved. Gently swish about ¼ of the cup in your mouth for 30 seconds. Make sure you force the water over the areas that feel sore. Then spit the water into the sink. Repeat until the entire cup is gone.

What about brushing with braces?

Here are some simple tips you can share with your child for the best results when brushing with braces on:

- Brush your teeth with a soft nylon toothbrush after you eat and before bed.

- Brush, rinse, and look; if you find any areas that are not clean, brush them again.

- Brush your gums as you brush your teeth (massage and stimulate).

- If no toothpaste is available, brush without.

- If you are unable to brush, rinse your mouth vigorously with water.

- Replace your old toothbrush when it gets worn out.

- It is absolutely essential that you continue regular visits to your family dentist for checkups and cleanings throughout your orthodontic treatment!

What type of foods should my child avoid while wearing braces?
There are four main types of food your child should avoid while wearing braces: **hard foods**, like ice, popcorn, peanut brittle, rock candy, and corn on the cob; **sticky foods,** like caramels, bubble gum, taffy, and suckers; **chewy foods,** like pizza crust, crusty breads, beef jerky, and gummy bears; and **sugary foods and drinks,** like cake, ice cream, cookies, pie, candy, and soda pop.

Why are retainers so important?
As we age, teeth naturally shift to the middle and crowd. Combined with late growth of the lower jaw, shifting of the teeth is expected following orthodontic treatment. Therefore, retainers are extremely important in the maintenance of your new smile following orthodontic treatment.

ABOUT THE AUTHOR

Robert F. Garrison, DMD, PA has more than 30 years of experience as an orthodontist. He works diligently to help patients achieve beautiful and healthy smiles through braces and a wide array of orthodontic treatments. A lifelong South Carolina resident, Dr. Garrison takes after his father who was a general dentist in Columbia, SC. Once he was old enough to choose his profession, he knew that he would be going into dentistry and ultimately decided that orthodontics was where he belonged. Starting his career in the Columbia and Lexington areas, he owned a successful orthodontic practice in Lexington for decades, where he put braces on more than 10,000 patients, including the daughter of former Governor of South Carolina and former United States Ambassador to the United Nations, Nikki Haley.

In 2016, Dr. Garrison sold his orthodontic practice in Lexington with the idea of retiring in Bluffton. However, it didn't take him long to realize that starting a new orthodontic practice made sense in so many ways. (Our passion never leaves us!) With his new practice well underway, Bluffton Orthodontics, Dr. Garrison is bringing his many years of experience and passion for orthodontics to the Lowcountry – creating a unique atmosphere that not only provides patients and families the highest quality of experienced orthodontic care and outstanding results, but offers a fun environment and stress-free journey to a beautiful smile.

A graduate of the University of South Carolina with a BS in Biology, he earned his Doctor of Medical Dentistry degree at the Medical University of South Carolina in Charleston and his degree in orthodontics from the Medical College of Georgia.

Aside from Dr. Garrison's amazing credentials, he is a member of the Southern Association of Orthodontists, American Association of Orthodontists, American Dental Association, SCAO (South Carolina Association of Orthodontics), and the South Carolina Dental Association. He offers a complimentary consultation and he and his team go above and beyond to cater to every individual need.

"Your smile is your best fashion accessory!"

Dr. Bob Garrison's story begins growing up with a father who was a family dentist. Being around him all the time, he quickly learned that his father genuinely enjoyed his profession, creating great working relationships not only with clientele but also with his staff. He loved and respected his dad's passion, empathy and unique interpersonal skills and always knew that he wanted to mirror his hero.

When he was a junior in dental school at the Medical University of South Carolina in Charleston, his father passed away. Needless to say, it was a heartbreaking time for him, but he also became suddenly aware that he would not be joining his dad's practice. He did some serious soul searching and decided to apply to the orthodontic residency program. He came to this realization remembering back to the time when he had braces as a teen. Not only was his life changed with a winning smile, but he remembered really liking his orthodontist and the fast-paced vigor of the office setting. He was fortunate to get selected at the Medical College of Georgia, who only accepts two residents per year. At the time, there was no orthodontic program in South Carolina, but he enthusiastically jumped right into his education in Georgia.

What is unique about Dr. Garrison's office?

Bluffton Orthodontics is a state-of-the-art office facility centrally located in Buckwalter Place, right next door to Station 300, where there's plenty of parking. They are both old school and high tech, meaning they offer highly personalized attention throughout your orthodontic journey, as well as the most advanced technologies. Their innovative technology includes CareStream3600 intraoral scans, which makes taking impressions faster and easier (and reduces the need for traditional impressions) by creating highly accurate digital 3D scans. They also offer a full range of digital x-rays and the most modern orthodontic appliances — leading to the most accurate diagnosis, effective treatments, and spectacular results. This office is truly open, bright, and comfortable.

Dr. Garrison and his team, including the office pedodontist, understand that their patients live busy lives and don't necessarily want to make an appointment during work, school, sports, or extra-curricular activities. That's why they offer extended appointment hours early in the morning, during lunch hours and evening appointments to accommodate anyone's schedule.

The team at Bluffton Orthodontics are all super caring, friendly and engaged people. They are constantly striving for ways to help every individual patient and pride themselves on giving patients the WOW factor. This unique team is thrilled to help you embrace your journey so you can leave with the most dazzling smile possible.

"We think it's important for employees to have fun... it drives employee engagement." –Tony Hsieh

From traditional to clear correct (an American-made product) to invisible to exclusive gold braces, Bluffton Orthodontics is so confident you'll love your experience with them, they back their services up with multiple guarantees! Dr. Garrison and his team's goal is your 100% satisfaction. If you are unsatisfied with the care you receive at any time during your treatment, simply let them know and they will do what it takes to make it right. That is their promise to you! They also proudly offer an affordability guarantee – keeping the prices fair, accepting most insurance plans, and offering customizable payment plans.

Aside from offering a welcoming and fun atmosphere, Bluffton Orthodontics is committed to offering high-quality orthodontic care to every person in The Lowcountry who needs it, including the Spanish-speaking community. Dr. Garrison truly wants to make your orthodontic care a seamless and comfortable process for everyone, and he provides a bilingual assistant to sit chairside with Spanish-speaking clients.

Bluffton Orthodontics delivers great customer service from start to finish and makes it their number one priority. Dr. Garrison conducts frequent staff meetings to assess and discuss any concerns, makes it a point to study and learn from what other successful entrepreneurs have done, listens intently to patients (and their loved ones!) and only employs the best staff available. In fact, the #1 reason that Dr. Garrison gets so many word-of-mouth referrals is due to his excellent customer service.

He also attributes his many referrals to his team who he says are caring, always willing to learn, always willing to change (they have a do-what-it-takes attitude), very excited about helping to grow the practice, and are basically just great people wanting to help patients, the community and the practice. In fact, this office cares about community immensely. The importance of giving back is a fundamental value for Dr. Garrison and his team at Bluffton Orthodontics, supporting their community regularly by donating resources and offering discounts. In recognition of the wonderful Beaufort and Jasper County School District Employees,

EMS and Fire Department members, and military families, Bluffton Orthodontics is happy to offer a discount on orthodontic treatments to all full-time employees, members, spouses, and their children.

Dr. Garrison believes that constantly keeping up with continuing education is extremely important and stays informed by attending seminars, reading journals, learning from online articles and hiring consultants to spend time in the office and advise. Over his many years of experience, he has learned much from other orthodontists and has been learning most recently from his new mentor, Dr. Dustin Burleson.

Dr. Garrison's favorite quote:
"Do unto others as you would have them do unto you."

When asked about his practice, he will tell you that he is 66 years young, feels energized and plans on working as long as it makes sense. His staff and patients give him a feeling of pride and his work gives his life meaning.

THE NEXT STEP:
Your Customized Smile Analysis

When you are ready, I urge you to schedule your **Customized Smile Analysis**, with a complimentary consultation; safe, digital x-rays (a $249 value) and exam; and report to you and your son or daughter—*all without cost or obligation.*

> Call us at 843-815-2521 or go to www.blufftonorthodontics.com to schedule your own Customized Smile Analysis.